Praise for

THE FIRST YEAR™

Hepatitis B

"Will Green describes from personal experience what it is like to live with chronic hepatitis B with knowledge, compassion, and just the right dash of humor. Everyone from patients and families to health care providers will truly benefit from reading *The First Year™—Hepatitis B*. This book fills a tremendous void and helps to bring hepatitis B out of the closet and into the light. Will Green's book is a wonderful gift to the hepatitis B community. Thank you!"

—JOAN M. BLOCK, R.N., BSN,
Co-Founder, Hepatitis B Foundation

"*The First Year™—Hepatitis B* is an amazing and impressive accomplishment. I like the fact that Will not only clarifies the emotional and physical stages of hep B, but he prioritizes this information so that you never feel overwhelmed by medical data. Every chronic condition needs a book like this. If your favorite liver doctor had an afternoon to shoot the breeze about hep B, you'd have what Will has gathered here. His writing is friendly, engaging, informative, warm, and supportive."

—R. TODD HARGAN, M.D.,
Northstar Medical Center, Chicago

"William Finley Green takes you on an innovative journey through the most difficult part of hepatitis B: enduring your first year. Having hep B can seem devastating and Will takes you on a discovery of facts, through the myths and fears, drawing from his rich personal experience. He makes you aware that living with this virus is synonymous with enjoying a near-normal life. The layout of the chapters is clear and includes current medical facts, practical ideas, and techniques that will enable you to harness your energy and cope with your condition. You will also learn how to apply your new knowledge to actual situations. Going through this book you realize that you have so much to do and look forward to, and it encourages you to do so."

—SHARAT C. MISRA, M.D., DM, FACG,
New Delhi, India

"This book is *exactly* what patients need. It *empowers* patients and is long overdue. Patients need to know that something *can* be done about their chronic condition, and it helps them ask the *right* questions of their doctors/nurses and take control of their own health. It gives patients, families, and all those who love a person with hepatitis B the tools to live as normal a life as possible. Doctors, nurses, and caregivers should read *The First Year™—Hepatitis B*, as it will give them a new perspective on patients not only with hepatitis B, but with chronic illness in general."

—PATRICE C. AL-SADEN, RN, CCRC,
Senior Clinical Research Coordinator—The Liver Center,
Harvard, Beth Israel Deaconess Medical Center, Boston

WILLIAM FINLEY GREEN is an artist, writer, and Italian translator. He has a degree in English from Oberlin College, and has spent ten years abroad in England, France, and Italy. He specializes in marketing, branding, and pharmaceutical translations for major multinational companies. Will was officially diagnosed with hepatitis B in 1993, but has been living with hepatitis since childhood. He lives in Chicago and Wisconsin.

THE COMPLETE FIRST YEAR™ SERIES

THE FIRST YEAR™

Hepatitis B

An Essential Guide for the Newly Diagnosed

William Finley Green

Foreword by Hari Conjeevaram, M.D.

MARLOWE & COMPANY ■ NEW YORK

THE FIRST YEAR™—*HEPATITIS B*
   An Essential Guide for the Newly Diagnosed
Copyright © 2002 by William Finley Green
Foreword copyright © 2002 by Hari Conjeevaram, M.D.

Published by
Marlowe & Company
An Imprint of Avalon Publishing Group Incorporated
161 William Street, 16th Floor
New York, NY 10038

The First Year™ and A Patient-Expert Walks You Through
   Everything You Need to Learn and Do™ are trade-
   marks of the Avalon Publishing Group.

Excerpt from *The Chronic Illness Experience* by Cheri
Register, copyright 1999, is reprinted by kind permission
of the Hazelden Foundation, Center City, Minnesota.

Library of Congress Cataloging-in-Publication Data
is available.

ISBN 1-56924-533-9

9 8 7 6 5 4 3 2 1

Designed by Pauline Neuwirth,
   Neuwirth and Associates, Inc.

Printed in the United States of America

Distributed by Publishers Group West

TO ALL THOSE
WHO WILLINGLY AND UNWILLINGLY
MAKE SENSE OF HBV

Contents

CONTENTS

Foreword

by Hari Conjeevaram, M.D.

HEPATITIS B (HBV) is one of the most intriguing and difficult viruses to understand, let alone attempt to write about. It also happens to be one of the most significant viruses that affect people and is carried by millions around the globe. If you've just been diagnosed with hepatitis B, you are definitely not alone.

Those new to the world of HBV inevitably feel overwhelmed by its lingo and its many faces and contradictions. Even those fascinated by it and who study it for years can get lost in its labyrinth. The wide range of clinical manifestations and the difficulty in treating people with HBV comes as a disappointment to the many who live with this virus. They feel amazed and saddened that so little attention is paid to a viral disease that touches so many others around the world. In the United States, attention is being greatly focused on another hepatitis virus, hepatitis C. We need to be aware that the equivalent of the entire population of the United States and Mexico has chronic hepatitis B worldwide, and that hepatitis B is the leading cause of liver cancer. It is ironic—yet sadly not a coincidence—that the word is just now getting out.

This dearth of information, understandably, can lead people with HBV to feel anxious. Through years of experience, we have come to realize that not everyone with HBV needs to be treated. However, it is very important for a person with HBV to learn about the virus and to be monitored on a regular basis. In my clinic, I start from the beginning and discuss the basics of HBV infection, starting with how one gets infected, the natural course of infection, diagnosing the infection, and all the available treatments. I try with simple language and a warm approach to help my patients learn more about their virus and what the different tests mean so they can better understand which stage of infection they are in. Over the years, I've learned that good teaching and good medicine rely on the same fundamental platform: the ability to explain complex issues with simple metaphors and a kind voice.

Usually I sit close to the patient and sketch a few diagrams about the hepatitis B virus and the various blood tests and clinical stages of infection. I also take them through the stages of a liver biopsy from mild hepatitis to severe hepatitis leading to cirrhosis. I want the patient to leave the clinic with a better understanding of the virus they are living with so they know to ask the right questions in the future. I firmly believe that knowing about one's HBV state lessens the anxiety and helps strip away the myths one may have been living with. As important as it is to learn about the fundamentals of hepatitis B, it is more important to know where one stands with his or her own infection. It is also important to realize that HBV affects people differently and is not associated with severe liver damage in everyone. And, in the end, we may not remember the list of medical terms or research studies involved, but we will remember a teacher or a doctor's subtle way of placing something into context with a knowing smile or a play on words.

The images in Will Green's book achieve just that: a virus that's an unwelcome guest raiding the liver cell's refrigerator, or the judges at an ice dancing championship trying to grade a biopsy. These images penetrate the mind and help us learn. And when we learn, we heal. When this happens we feel empowered, and we are better able to take care of our bodies and our spirits.

I have always hoped that someone with HBV would write a book about his or her life with it. In addition to offering a different perspective, *The First Year™—Hepatitis B* underscores the importance of the patient's role in educating not only himself but the millions of others living with this virus. I commend Will for taking on this challenge, but more importantly, for taking it an extra step and seeing that it was done right. His passion to learn, educate, inspire, and help others like him is felt throughout this book. Will humanizes HBV by making it three-dimensional, and he helps you learn just enough about HBV to build a platform upon which you can put everything into perspective. Every day we're bombarded by data: anyone can read medical journals, see a video of a liver biopsy on the Internet, or share stories in online support groups. But often we don't know how to process this information or place it into context. *The First Year™—Hepatitis B* does this effortlessly. I wish I'd had this book to give the multitude of HBV patients that I've seen over the past ten years of my career as a hepatologist.

Patient-written guides have traditionally had a bad reputation among medical professionals. But now we are seeing a new breed of author/patient—authors who have not only made sense of their own personal experience with a disease but have stepped back far enough from their experience to objectify it, making it informative and helpful to other patients without a trace of self-indulgence. As one reads through this book, it is obvious that Will has done his homework. Having experienced HBV firsthand, he navigates the fine line between what you need to know now and what you can learn next week or next month. His book draws you step-by-step into the remarkable story of hepatitis B and its idiosyncratic personality, making it seem less foreboding and more familiar. His discussion of diet, interpersonal issues, and exercise should be read by anyone with any kind of hepatitis. This book demystifies and destigmatizes the disease, making it a must-read not only for those with the virus, but their friends, families, and colleagues. For any doctor, nurse, or physician's assistant who works with those with HBV, this book is essential, affording them a whole new perspective on the most important person: the patient.

Will offers a balanced, nonjudgmental, and expanded definition of healing that anchors us in the concrete: taking responsibility for yourself and your treatment, staying curious, having fun, opening your heart and mind, sharing with others, listening to your spirit, and taking nothing for granted. Those are all very powerful antidotes.

HARI CONJEEVARAM, M.D. is a hepatologist with the University of Michigan. He lives in Ann Arbor, Michigan.

Introduction

Roughly 150,000 new hepatitis B infections occur each year in the United States, and an estimated 1.5 million Americans are chronic carriers of the hepatitis B virus.

One in 20 people in the United States will get hepatitis B some time during their lives, while two thirds of the world's population has been infected with HBV at some time in their lives.

The estimated global prevalence of chronic HBV infection is 350 million individuals, or about 5 percent of the world's population.

Hepatitis B causes 83 percent of all of instances of liver cancer, and is the ninth leading cause of death worldwide. One million people worldwide die from HBV complications every year.

WORLD HEALTH ORGANIZATION STATISTICS

YOU TRIED to donate blood and got a call from the blood bank or health department. Maybe you're pregnant and had to do some routine blood tests. Or your mother was recently diagnosed with hepatitis B (HBV) so her doctor suggested the whole family be tested. Perhaps you've been feeling tired. You can't seem to shake that bout of flu that you had a few months back. Your doctor ran a series of tests a week or so ago, and you've returned for a follow-up visit or have received a phone call from the nurse.

Then you get the news. And you feel that somehow you'll never experience life quite the same way again.

Whether you have an acute (recent infection lasting up to six months) or chronic (more than six months duration) case of hepatitis B, the information in this book will apply to you. If you're diagnosed as acute, your blood will be tested again in a few months to see if the virus is still in your blood. This book will help you through these anxious next few months and help you manage your expectations about the future. If you've been diagnosed as chronic, however, you've probably just received your *second* call after subsequent blood tests. Fortunately, less than 10 percent of adults who come into contact with HBV develop chronic hepatitis B, but the younger you are at the time of infection, the more likely it is that you will become chronic. Infants are especially at risk for developing chronic infection.

When you've been diagnosed with HBV, you learn something about unadulterated fear and pure panic. This is your poorly timed and unwelcome initiation. But here's the good news: very few (around 1 percent) of us develop acute fulminant (life-threatening) hepatitis B. And knowing that you carry the virus is far better than being in the dark, as you can take care of your body, alter your diet, monitor your liver function, and try to rid your body of the virus or at least lower your viral load with medication. Ignorance is decidedly not bliss when you have this virus.

Although today HBV may seem as threatening as a rattlesnake about to strike, thinking of it as a shadow that follows you is a more accurate metaphor for HBV carriers, at least in the initial stage. Although it's always there, sometimes you notice it often and sometimes, thankfully, you don't notice it at all.

Those of us with hepatitis B have no magic solution. We face a seemingly endless series of hurdles. Information, especially for those without access to the Internet, is hard to come by. Once we manage to find information, we must learn how to separate the good data from the bad. Then we have to find a doctor who knows and/or cares as much as we do about HBV, and despite new, more effective treatments, many doctors we put our faith in choose not to treat HBV because that is what they were taught years ago.

Promising treatments are on the horizon and we desperately need to stay informed. Only when we have information and a doctor in place can we concentrate on the considerable task of treating our bodies, minds, and spirits.

Despite the fact that a vaccine has been available for hepatitis B since 1982, it wasn't widely administered until the 1990s. Numerous and unwarranted urban legends circulate about the HBV vaccine's safety, particularly for children. This is unfortunate, particularly when children are the most vulnerable targets for chronic HBV. No less than 95 percent of children age two or younger become chronic if infected with the HBV. Despite the vaccine's availability and relatively low cost, more than 150,000 new cases of hepatitis B surface each year in America, and many more of us unknowingly harbor the virus of what is sometimes called the silent killer.

Sixty-four percent of all cases of HBV could have been prevented had vaccines been offered and administered, according to Dr. Miriam Alter, speaking at the 2000 "Management of HBV" Conference at the National Institute of Health. And a recent survey of gay men discovered that only 9 percent are vaccinated against the disease. Few things can be more frustrating than contracting a disease for which a vaccine is available.

Since it is likely that the virus can go unnoticed for decades, we who were not vaccinated as children are only now discovering in adulthood that the virus has gone undetected and has done damage to our livers. In fact, those of us who are in our twenties or older have a greater likelihood of harboring the disease if we were never vaccinated. Thus, despite the existence of a safe and effective vaccine, statistics report a consistent increase in hospital admissions and deaths due to hepatitis B.

What happened to me

I had HBV for as many as twenty-five years before I was diagnosed. Seven years ago work-related chemical poisoning left me bedridden. My skin had a blue cast and I had circles under my eyes like bruises. I felt heavy, as if hot lead coursed through my veins and concrete weighed in my stomach. In retrospect, I can decipher that most of the symptoms I was experiencing were induced by the chemicals I had inhaled on the job, while just a few were due to my scarred liver which was particularly susceptible to those fumes. After six months of tests, my primary physician called me in: "Well, I think we've finally got an answer here," he said, with a combined look of indifference and relief, without any explanation, and certainly without compassion: "You've got chronic hepatitis B, which isn't that bad, but you may need a transplant when you're older. We don't treat it. Nothing to worry about—just don't drink any alcohol."

Somehow I managed to get home. After a flurry of calls, I tracked down a copy of my childhood medical chart and discovered that I had elevated enzymes when I was 11. The doctor had written "smoldering hepatitis" in the margin of my test results. Suddenly, it was clear why I had had recurring periods of severe fatigue and an assortment of unpleasant symptoms over the years. It took years for me to realize just how incomplete and misleading the doctor's words were.

After years of practicing safe sex and avoiding drugs and alcohol, I found myself with chronic hepatitis B. How could that be? I was so weak I had to sit and take a break after climbing the first landing in my apartment building. I thought over the doctor's message. Something didn't ring true. If it wasn't so bad, why was I so incapacitated? Why did I look and feel so terrible? If it wasn't so bad, why were my enzymes so high? Why couldn't I concentrate or remember names? And why would I ever need a liver transplant?

I decided to be proactive. I went out to find a book about hepatitis B. The local library had nothing. Then I went to several bookstores. Nothing. It felt like a conspiracy. There were a few about hepatitis C—but none for B? I imagined the bookstores had sold out. After all, the total number of those with hepatitis B in the world outnumbers those with hepatitis C by roughly 10 to 1. Perhaps the books on hepatitis C were useful for those diagnosed with hepatitis B? I was confused and felt alone.

I looked online and found several good resources. My rather steep learning curve began. I surfed and sifted through a wide variety of sites from dry and oblique official sites that seemed to have more information about the organization itself and fundraising drives than the actual disease, to personal homepages with excellent firsthand experiences but a paucity of hard facts and trustworthy statistics. Although I had bookmarked dozens of sites, I still felt lost. No one could prepare me for the trials and tribulations of the HBV experience I was about to embark upon.

In the meantime, after finding a new specialist, I started treatment. Fortunately, my blood work after the first three months of taking the medication Lamivudine showed that my virus count had gone from 5.7 million per unit to a mere 200. Through the cell phone I heard the tiny metallic voice of the nurse say "Isn't that great? You should be cheering! Hello?" I was very close to reaching my goal of total or near-total suppression of the virus that had entered my bloodstream and threatened to take over my life. I felt like I'd won the lottery.

Four doctors and six years later, I'm glad to say I'm feeling good. So good, in fact, I fear I've become an infomercial: "Hi! I'm Will! I lift weights and run along the lake! No more fatigue!" The truth is, however, that my well-being was hard won. And it doesn't always last for long. Since my childhood years, hepatitis B has damaged my liver and left me with stage 3 fibrosis. I'm trying to head cirrhosis off at the pass. I'd really like to keep the liver I was born with. And I'd also like to help you avoid getting to this place.

Where the focus is

I've written this book to answer questions and provide insights for a reader who resembles the person I was six years ago, with my head propped up on my hands in front of a monitor, desperately looking for a piece of good advice about HBV and an understanding ear. For this reason, I not only talk about diagnostic and treatment processes, but I also discuss how this disease affects your mind, your sense of self, and your relationships with family, friends, and coworkers.

The result is a book that is centered on the individual person, organized not as a cold encyclopedic listing of medical terms, but tailored to the phases and circumstances that a person with HBV encounters—from the initial discovery of the virus in your bloodstream to the first biopsy, from initial treatments to social situations and starting a family.

The information in this book is broken down into explanations of the core issues you face at each step of your treatment, starting with the facts you need to know immediately and then gradually giving you the details you'll find useful further ahead. Some information will be mentioned briefly and then expanded and reinforced in subsequent chapters. Diet, exercise, alternative treatments, and the latest developments in traditional Western medicine are covered, in addition to frank discussions about navigating social situations or negotiating personal issues.

Instead of weighing you down with dozens of statistics and research reports about HBV treatments that may be outdated by the time you read this book, I have chosen to focus on helping you build a solid foundation of knowledge about the disease from which to make informed decisions that affect your health.

How to use this book

Given that the organization of this book is tailored to your situational dynamic and the assumption that you've come straight to the bookstore after your diagnosis, you may assume that you should skip ahead to "more advanced" chapters if you've been living with HBV for more than a few years. I recommend that you begin at the beginning and read day by day. There is so much to learn about HBV that we can all use a little pep talk and a refresher course on HBV tactics and truths.

Each day, week, or month in this book is divided into a *Living* and a *Learning* section. The *Living* section deals with the problem of living with this chronic disease. After speaking to many people with HBV, I found that we all have looked for someone to tell us how it feels from an emotional—rather than merely physical or statistical—perspective. Of course we want to know what HBV is going to do to our livers, but we also want to know how it is going to affect our lives. Therefore, the *Living* sections strive to make you feel that you are not alone and that what you're experiencing is normal. The *Learning* sections aim for the left side of your brain—the side that is hungry for data, statistics, and pure science. I hope to engage both hemispheres.

You'll notice I have included a few comments from real people with HBV and their families. Some of their names have been altered and some of their comments have been abridged. I have included firsthand observations that may or may not resonate with your experience. Regardless, I believe that listening to others' voices will help us find ours.

Terms in **boldface** are defined in the glossary at the end of the book.

I will not prescribe

After years of complaining about a lack of resources, I decided to stop whining and start writing. Let me say up front: I don't belong to any voluntary societies, I don't run my own HBV website, I haven't appeared on any talk shows or in videos, and I haven't done any published research or consulted for any large pharmaceutical companies. I don't have any "official" qualifications except more than 20 years of living with hepatitis B and a decade of writing and translation experience, much of it in the pharmaceutical field. I have lived through this experience and taken notes along the way, and I have an intimate knowledge of what it means to get up every morning despite chronic fatigue, irritable bowels, and aches.

Since I am not a doctor, I will not prescribe for you in this book. Although I will supply you with extensive information about various treatments, diet, and exercise, I will not make a value judgment about which is best for you. The information in this book has been found to be useful for other people with HBV. It is up to you, though, in partnership with your doctor and other health care practitioners, to decide your own strategy for living with HBV.

What you will read here are various experiences—good and bad—about every aspect of living with HBV, and these will give you a solid foundation for deciding what approach might work for you. There are new and exciting treatments coming our way, and much of the treatment information in this book will require periodic updates. My goal is to empower you with adequate and pertinent background information which, when combined with your thirst for knowledge, will serve you well in the coming months and years.

Keep on learning, keep on growing

In the chapters that follow, I hope to guide you in finding comfort and strength by informing you not only about HBV and current treatments, but also about how you can take an active and constructive role in your treatment and your day-to-day coexistence with the virus. Numerous factors will determine what parts of this book will be most useful to you: how long the virus has been residing in your body, how strong your constitution is, how many frozen margaritas or bacon cheeseburgers you've consumed or cigarettes you've smoked, whether you work in a factory or on a farm, how stressful your life is overall. We don't care how you got HBV, though you may find yourself faced with ignorance in that regard from others who are less understanding.

I hope that this book will help you negotiate a "peaceful coexistence" with the virus, whether it is in your bloodstream or that of a family member or friend. Remember, you have HBV "cousins" all over the world (400 million) who understand what you're going through.

Take a deep breath and read on. I'm honored that you've chosen this book. You've taken a great first step in your resolve to learn as much as you can about your body and HBV.

Condemned To . . .
Taking Care of Yourself

ALTHOUGH THERE are as many possible ways of react-
ing to a new diagnosis as there are newly diagnosed patients,
psychiatrists have inventoried the familiar yet difficult passages
we make towards grief and adjusting to loss: denial, anger, bar-
gaining, depression, and acceptance. We can all look at a calendar and chart the weeks that we experience each of these
emotions, although they may not occur in that order, and they
may loop.

In the HBV Internet support group I have belonged to for
the past few years (see Day 4) Sheree and Steve, founders and
moderators of the group, usually respond to a new member with
the phrase "glad you found us, sorry you had to find us." We
who have made the journey from initial shock to final acceptance know that you face many challenges, but thankfully we
also know that in time you will unearth hidden opportunities for
self-knowledge.

While this may seem hard to believe today as you and your
family race to understand the scope of the disease and how it
will affect your lives, eventually you will be able to comprehend
the full effect of HBV on your body and psyche. It's common
to feel like you have lost control over your life and your body;
however, you will slowly learn to take control and make bold,

important choices. At its best, learning to live with HBV is a journey towards self-discovery.

Managing stress and anxiety is critical

Managing your life with HBV often involves learning to manage your feelings and your energy. Since the times of the ancient poets a spiritual condition has been made out of a simple biological imbalance, and the study of melancholy is perhaps one of the few true instances where medicine, art, and philosophy converge. In fact, the word "melancholy" has its etymological roots in the dark **bile** that is responsible, in part, for our malaise.

When your liver is challenged, stress and anxiety can pull you down both emotionally and physically. From this moment, you will start developing new muscles for dealing with chronic illness. What you do today will set the tone for the years ahead. Your first impulse may be to talk at length with your family. Or perhaps you will want to be alone. Do not expect to make sense of HBV today. Rather, express your feelings in ways that do not hurt you or your liver. Choose a good listener. Select someone you know who has had a life-threatening or chronic illness. If you can't find this person in your home, your town, or in your address book, call a professional therapist who has experience dealing with chronic illness, and make an appointment. Don't be ashamed to let it all out.

Why is this so important? As you will find throughout the coming months and years, you will need to be attentive to your feelings, especially stressors. If you've been putting off dealing directly and effectively with stress in your life until now, a diagnosis is a euphemistic shovel on the forehead. We have to become aware and responsible when it comes to managing our emotions. For many of us, especially those with fibrosis and cirrhosis, a particularly stressful day at work or even a seemingly insignificant disagreement can bring on moderate—even severe—fatigue.

Feeling down is normal

Not surprisingly, many people with HBV experience depression. As if news of the **virus** and occasionally feeling like a leper isn't enough, we also have to deal with HBV's effect on our ability to think clearly and positively. Putting up with daily fatigue or itching can sometimes put a real damper on enjoying life. And not being able to down a cold beer and a pizza with our old friends may make us want to avoid socializing altogether. Many of us with HBV express feelings of loneliness and estrangement. Isolation can be a ramp to depression.

It is not a mystical process. We simply may not have the energy to keep up. Our livers don't always allow our minds to fully function, so sometimes we can't tell what is emotional or psychological from what is induced physically. This makes it even more difficult to separate the wheat from the chaff. However, we need to deal directly and actively with our emotions and be courageous enough to admit needing a therapist. Sometimes even treatment can be a direct cause of depression. Trying to be an HBV martyr won't get you very far. Speak your mind. Ask for help.

You are in the driver's seat

You may feel today that you've been robbed of basic freedoms. You may feel like your self-image is evaporating. You may feel that you did not deserve this diagnosis. You might direct anger at God or perhaps the person who infected you with this virus, or you may feel that your life is suddenly spinning out of control. This is only natural. You need not feel guilty or worried about harboring these feelings. You have plenty of time to get a hold of yourself, and it will take time until you feel like you can integrate HBV into your everyday existence, recognizing that you have just as much control over and choice for your future as you always have.

Cheri Register, in her insightful and beautifully written book *The Chronic Illness Experience*, provides the following parameters for identifying how we will choose to fit into the spectrum from perfectly healthy to hopelessly ill:

- You can tough it out, ignoring symptoms at the risk of getting worse, or you can check out every little quirk, at the risk of hypochondria.
- You can shop for miracle cures, at the risk of harming yourself, or you can trust one doctor's judgment, at the risk of selecting unwisely.
- You can keep your ailment secret, at the risk of deception, or you can talk openly about it, at the risk of self-pity.
- You can ask friends for help, at the risk of becoming a burden, or you can hold fast to your independence, at the risk of isolation.
- You can insist that your family treats you as normal and healthy, at the risk of denying them release for their own worries about you, or you can let them protect you, at the risk of becoming dependent and childlike.
- You can strain your body to the limit, at the risk of harming yourself, or you can play it safe, at the risk of becoming an invalid.

○ You can live in terror of degeneration and death, at the risk of becoming immobilized, or you can look upon each good day as a special dispensation, at the risk of smugness.

○ You can insist on controlling the course of your life, at the risk of frustration, or you can go with the flow, at the risk of passivity.

○ You can be angry about your fate, at the risk of bitterness, or you can focus on your blessings, at the risk of self-delusion.

No one can say with absolute certainty which of these extremes is the healthier or exactly where the healthy medium lies. Only trial and error will reveal the most livable choice.

Taking a deep breath: the chronic experience

What is the chronic experience all about, then? It's about having to reevaluate yourself and your priorities. It involves the seemingly contradictory traits of learning how to let go while taking on greater responsibility for decisions that you face. It's about managing and harnessing a decreased supply of energy. It's thinking about your body in a new way, about the art of maintaining self-esteem while you're contagious, about savoring beautiful moments, and learning how to pay attention. It's about having to divulge your private life to strangers, acquaintances, and institutions, and how they'll adapt their thinking about and/or treatment of you. Finally, it is about how to care for your body and your mind as if caring was an undiscovered world.

Our world likes facile categorization: we're labeled as "sick" in a healthy world. However, studies show that nearly half of the American population suffers from at least one chronic condition; anything from chronic fatigue to heart disease, while many more suffer from multiple chronic diseases. In my opinion, it would be more constructive to create new categories which more closely reflect reality, such as: "healthy with a chronic condition" and "healthy without a chronic condition—*yet*." Does being sick still have to have a stigma attached to it as if it were an unnatural part of life?

Finally, and most importantly, there is a never-ending list of viruses that thrive on humans. HBV is just one of the most popular and persistent. HBV is, in fact, a natural occurrence and it has been around for centuries. Don't be ashamed of your virus, and don't allow others to treat your hepatitis B virus differently that any other virus. Everyone has viruses of some kind. There is no room for value judgments or viral discrimination. Stand tall. Be proud.

IN A SENTENCE:

> *You have the freedom to choose how your life will be with HBV because you can proactively manage your energy, diet, treatment, and feelings.*

learning

Being and Feeling Contagious—Common First Day Questions

Entering the world of HBV

HEPATITIS B is an extraordinarily complex disease to describe or explain. The various **genotypes**, degrees of infection, widely varying strategies for treatment, and even the names and acronyms of tests for which you've just given blood are unnecessarily confusing. Your results will often not stay stable, performing what we call flip-flops. In addition, tests performed in different countries use different parameters for measuring results, causing further confusion for those of us who switch doctors, travel, or live abroad. HBV also behaves differently from other viruses, and at times it seems to defy logic.

Further confusion is due to the fact that HBV names and acronyms are so similar that even physicians sometimes mix them up. A global standardization of terms, units of measurement, and grading scales is probably on the horizon. We can only hope so.

In the meantime, keep a cheat sheet (see Resources) on hand to make sure that you're remembering these HBV-related terms correctly. The hepatitis alphabet extends from A to G, and each virus behaves differently and requires different attention. Some of us are **co-infected**, meaning we have more than one type of virus in our blood. For example, some of us have both **HIV** and HBV. It is even more confusing that there are mutations of the virus and different HBV geno-types, and that these genotypes also, by chance, range from A to G.

The following chapters will inform you about tests and various stages and strains of hepatitis, and will provide explanations of their importance in gauging your health and potential treatment.

First Day Questions

For starters, here are the most commonly asked questions (and answers) from those who have just been diagnosed.

How come I had no idea? When did I get this?

HBV is disturbingly contagious. The mind boggles when it tries to digest the fact that HBV is 100 times more infectious than HIV. The virus can live for at least one week outside the body on a dry surface. One in 20 Americans has been infected with the virus at some point in their lives. Statistics tell us that up to 40 percent of us have no idea where we got it, and knowing where it came from will not change how this disease will affect us. You have come into contact with the virus via blood (by sharing a needle, razor, or straw used for snorting drugs; getting a tattoo or piercing; receiving a transfusion, undergoing surgery in the operating room, or having work done in the dentist's chair) or bodily fluid through sexual contact. Many of us have been infected at birth by our mothers.

The American Liver Foundation says that an estimated 40 percent of the people who are infected with HBV (**acute** or **chronic**) have no noticeable symptoms. Although there are ten times as many HBV+ patients as HIV+ patients worldwide, doctors rarely order hepatitis blood tests if none of the symptoms are present. Even worse, studies have also shown that not even patients with elevated **enzymes** receive adequate follow-up attention. Hopefully this situation will change, as more information is made available about HBV and its daunting demographics.

Why have I never heard of it before?
Why wasn't I given the vaccine?

Until recently, there hasn't been much information circulating about HBV. There wasn't even a single English-language book on the market geared to people with HBV. Despite increasing worldwide numbers (10 people with HBV for every 1 with HIV), HBV receives less than 1 percent of the funding that HIV research does. A few well-known personalities have helped get the word out about hepatitis C (country singer Naomi Judd is one), but little press has been given to hepatitis B.

This is unfortunate, especially since a **vaccine** for HBV has been available since 1982. Clearly, more primary physicians should have recommended that their patients be given the vaccine, and more politicians and health officials should have required that schoolchildren get the vaccine. We can all be proactive in this regard. We can encourage our friends and colleagues and their children to be vaccinated, and we can write letters to our politicians, encouraging them to make the vaccine compulsory in our schools. Although childhood HBV vaccination is now mandatory in 43 states, most states only approved this requirement in the past few years. A recent survey by the American College Health Association found that very few college students had received the HBV vaccine, despite the fact that 75 percent of new HBV infections occur between the ages of 15 and 39. We can voice our disappointment with our physicians and encourage them to be more vigilant and informed with regard to HBV.

You may have already had HBV when you got the vaccine. Some were vaccinated years ago without having had their blood checked for HBV beforehand. If we have the virus in our system already, the vaccine most likely has no effect whatsoever.

A silent giant, the liver is the largest organ in your body. It is well-behaved, hard working, and extraordinarily efficient. One possible reason that HBV is not as high profile as other viruses or diseases, perhaps, is the liver doesn't call attention to itself in the way that our hearts, lungs, and stomachs do. Since it feels no pain the liver has no chance to complain. And, despite enormous responsibilities, it carries out its tasks silently and effectively.

Another reason why HBV is underpublicized is that it most often strikes the poor populations of Third World countries, and that, unfortunately, doesn't make it glamorous or trendy. Until a famous actor, athlete, or model gets HBV, it won't be an exciting story for the media.

AM I CONTAGIOUS?

If your blood tests show a high level of HBV (this is your **viral load**) and you are **'e' antigen** positive, you are *very contagious*.

If your tests show that you are 'e' antigen negative with a detectable amount of virus in your blood (more on this in Day 2), it is likely that you are contagious.

If your tests show that you are 'e' antigen negative with an undetectable amount of virus, you are probably not contagious, but there is still a small chance that you are infectious to some degree.

While there is a vaccine for hepatitis B, it is also necessary to use universal precautions when dealing with potentially infected materials. Often, people infected with hepatitis B or HIV do not know they are infected. It is impossible to know just by looking whether or not someone is infected with a blood-borne disease. Therefore you need to treat all blood and body fluids as if they may be contaminated. Never reuse syringes or acupuncture or tattooing needles. Do not clean up broken glass with your fingers—use a brush and dustpan instead—and never dispose of it in a regular trash bag where custodians could get cut when emptying the trash. Disinfect potentially contaminated materials and surfaces with a 10 percent bleach solution. Make sure you don't splash blood or contaminated body fluids into eyes, cuts, sores, or open lesions. If you do contact someone else's blood, wash quickly and thoroughly with soap and water.

By following these simple precautions, you can protect yourself from all blood-borne **pathogens**, not just hepatitis B.

WILL I DIE FROM THIS?

Although your prognosis will depend on many factors such as age at time of infection, diet, treatment, etc., here are the cold numbers from research institutes: Out of 100 people infected with HBV, only five to ten will become chronic. HBV will lead to **cirrhosis** (severe scarring) in 25 percent of those persons who become chronic. HBV can also lead to liver cancer, but the rate varies widely depending on your race and the continent you call home. For example, studies show that 15 percent of Asians with chronic HBV develop HCC (**hepatocellular carcinoma**, or liver cancer) over time. HBV has the dubious honor of being the leading cause of liver cancer in the world.

To sum up, chances are quite favorable that you will not die from complications due to HBV. But your chances will be improved by regular visits to your specialist (even if you feel good), periodic testing, and by making personal adjustments based on the diet, exercise, and stress-relief ideas offered in this book.

I FEEL FINE. WHY SHOULD I BE CONCERNED?

It is very important to remember that *how you feel at any given time does not necessarily correspond to the actual condition of your liver*. There are too many other variables to consider, and you should never assume anything until you have blood test results and, when performed, a **biopsy** report in your hand.

Some of us have no symptoms despite the presence of severe scarring (**fibrosis**), while others have many intense symptoms though no damage whatsoever. With so many variables in play (viral load, liver enzymes, diet, mood, environmental factors), only a liver biopsy can truly gauge the actual condition of your liver. You may be asked to have a biopsy particularly if your liver enzymes are elevated. A liver biopsy is a good way to minimize the chance that you will develop complications of cirrhosis and die from liver disease because it effectively and objectively gauges your liver's health on a cellular level and may provide enough information to help you avoid developing severe liver disease.

WHAT DO I NEED TO DO RIGHT AWAY?

Your partner and/or those who share your home should check to see if they have received the vaccine or have had HBV in the past and recovered from it. If not, they should be tested for HBV and get the vaccination.

You should not share razors, earrings, needles, or toothbrushes. Traces of blood can even be detected on nail clippers or other manicure tools. Some experts even go as far as to recommend that you don't share hairbrushes or combs given that scabs on the scalp can bleed.

If you have gingivitis, or bleeding from the gums, you might want to brush early in the morning if you have plans for a romantic evening to minimize the presence of trace amounts of blood in your saliva. If you bite your lip you may want to wait a day before kissing someone who doesn't have HBV antibodies. Be careful about menstrual blood as well. If you cut yourself and leave traces of blood, use a household cleaner that contains bleach or a mixture of bleach and water to clean the surfaces, since HBV can live for a least a week outside of the body.

Pregnant women should be extra careful to monitor their health, considering that they can pass the virus to their babies. About one in every 500 to 1,000 pregnant women has hepatitis worldwide. If a pregnant mother is HBeAg negative, chances are less than 10 percent that her baby will get the virus if not vaccinated after birth. However, there is up to an 80–90 percent chance her baby will be infected if she is HBeAg positive and the baby has not been vaccinated. See Month 5 for more information on pregnancy and HBV.

Ask your doctor to give you the HAV (hepatitis A virus) vaccine as soon as possible if you haven't already received it, since co-infection with HAV can be very dangerous for those with HBV.

You will need to stop drinking alcohol, and inform your doctor about any medications or herbal supplements you are taking. Some can harm your liver or have a negative effect on your treatment.

And remember to find a good listener. My best listeners have been friends with HIV or cancer—they can empathize. If you aren't yet prepared to tell friends or family and can afford it, call a professional therapist with chronic illness experience and make an appointment. If you don't have insurance and live in a larger metropolitan area, you may be able to find a therapy clinic that charges on a sliding scale according to income.

Do I REALLY HAVE TO STOP DRINKING ALCOHOL?

Yes, really. Today, in fact. Alcohol is highly toxic to the HBV liver even in moderation, and over time can lead to severe and irreparable scarring, otherwise know as cirrhosis. If your liver becomes cirrhotic, it cannot regenerate. Also, do not consume alcohol if you're taking acetaminophen or paracetamol. This even applies to those without HBV.

Not ever being able to enjoy an alcoholic beverage seems like an unnecessary inconvenience, especially if you feel fine, given that much socializing is anchored in the consumption of alcohol. My passion for fine Italian red wine, for example, was immediately shelved. I don't regret giving it up. In order to avoid alienating myself from others at important occasions, I occasionally let a waiter pour just 'a finger' of Chianti so I can still raise a glass in toast and enjoy the bouquet. Others choose to enjoy a half glass of wine or champagne only during the holidays.

While you're at it, try to quit smoking. As a 15-year veteran smoker of strong Italian cigarettes, I can testify that tar and nicotine do your liver no favors. Joint aches, back pain, and fatigue will probably increase if you're smoking. Of course you will also smell like an ashtray and look terrible. Studies show that smoking also increases your chance of getting liver cancer by up to 3 percent, as if lung cancer and heart disesase weren't enough reasons to make you think twice.

Reality check: putting it into perspective

Is HBV a condemnation? It may feel that way today since you're probably still in crisis mode. However, as the years go by and you adapt, modify, and improve your daily regimen, you may eventually consider living with HBV as simply being "condemned" to taking care of yourself physically and emotionally. Living with HBV requires many adjustments, yet all of them are manageable when you phase them in slowly. And they also happen to be quite good for you.

The longer we live with HBV, the longer we find that diet, along with exercise, is the key to minimizing the most common HBV symptoms. The nutrition chapters in the book will show you how to find satisfying substitutions, develop simple menus, and creatively avoid fast food. You will undoubtedly develop an appetite for refining and improving your own habits and rhythms, and will look back at your past life—the one where you ate chili cheese dogs and nachos and threw back shots of Jäegermeister— with appalled amusement.

IN A SENTENCE:

> *HBV may feel like a condemnation today, but the reality is that you must take care of yourself and your loved ones both physically and emotionally.*

The Day After— Common Reactions

PEOPLE REACT in many ways to a diagnosis of HBV. For some it doesn't register for months or even years. Others react immediately, fueled by fear and trepidation. Here are a few of the most common reactions, though it is possible to experience a combination of these reactions.

Reaction: Joy

Believe it or not, sometimes getting a diagnosis is a cause for joy. You feel like a bit of light has finally been shed on your condition. You feel a sense of renewal after a long period of darkness, aching, and fatigue. For years you may have been accused of being a hypochondriac or a whiner. Your partner probably kept silent about it, but deep down he or she may have believed you were born that way, complaining to whoever was nearby and being a baby—trading aches for attention. Or your mother probably thought you didn't eat well enough and accused you of burning your candle at both ends. Colleagues almost certainly thought you took a few too many sick days.

A few among us experience an enormous sense of relief when a blood test finally gives a name to our malaise. It can be particularly gratifying to validate our intuition. Our family may think this is our peculiar way of dealing with grief, or that the news has affected us psychologically more than we know, that our giddiness is really a kind of inverted shock, a warning sign that we're about to crash and burn.

Out of desperation we self-diagnose, entertaining a wide range of dark scenarios. Initially we may pass it off as mono or the flu, or in the words of my gray-haired childhood doctor, "a difficult puberty." If we read up on it and have a few more years of searching under our belts, we may ascribe symptoms to allergies, low blood sugar, chronic depression, diabetes, chronic fatigue syndrome, or anemia. More difficult or acute symptoms may have forced us to consider dramatic prospects like cancer, for example. Did people around us think we were crazy? Probably. Did we ever doubt ourselves? Probably not. Sometimes the body just knows.

Reaction: Denial

HBV doesn't usually show. Most of us have no outward symptoms of infection whatsoever. Although some still think that **jaundice** (yellowing of the skin and eyes) is a telltale sign, it seldom occurs in those who have chronic HBV without cirrhosis.

Looking good on the outside makes it all the more likely and logical—in a rather perverse way—that you will willfully and magically change your diagnosis to HBV negative. If you must insist, eliminate any last doubt by having the doctor retest you. And have your support group and **hepatologist** help you interpret the tests. There have been instances over the years where primary physicians (including mine) misinterpreted initial tests. There have also been a few instances where tests contradicted one another or showed a false positive result. That is the HBV equivalent of winning the lottery.

Unfortunately, chances are crushingly good that there were no mistakes. Remember: denial about the virus can be even more harmful than the virus itself.

Reaction: Anger

If someone knowingly put you at risk and has infected you, anger is a fair and warranted reaction. Warranted doesn't translate to healthy, so working through this anger now is wise, either with a therapist or a good listener. If someone has unknowingly put you at risk, anger is probably a waste of time. Your liver would rather you let go and move on. Focus on your health, not on the past. If you've been infected by a transfusion, dentist or doctor, or tattoo parlor that did not use universal precautions, call your local health department.

However, if you're someone who hasn't ever knowingly come into contact with disease via a friend, family member, or sexual partner, being diagnosed can seem especially unfair. Life puts us into contact with an interminable array of problems and challenges. Bacteria and viruses are just a doorknob away. The universe is expanding and viruses are adapting and mutating. Things change. Unfortunately, our bodies are vulnerable and susceptible to life. We have to be nimble and adapt. We have to accept. HBV will teach you all of this.

If your infection is entirely your doing, don't beat yourself up. It's not your fault the virus is 100 times more infectious than HIV. It doesn't take a lot of talent to get it. Here's how Pamela puts it: "A few of us become trapped in trying to figure out where we got the virus, as though that information could somehow make us better. Like we could undo it if we knew where it came from. In my opinion, this is a sidetrack, and one that can be a source of irresolvable anger for some people."

Reaction: Panic

I panicked on the day of my diagnosis. I didn't feel like I was up to facing the challenge that the disease presented, and I remember feeling that my head was about to explode. I felt like I couldn't breathe.

Panic calls for taking quick measures. If you're panicking today, turn to the exercise section of Week 4 and read the breathing exercises chapter very carefully. Take a hot shower or bath. Afterwards, climb on your bed, turn down the light or put on some of your favorite music, and do these breathing exercises for 15 minutes. Then come back to this book. If this sounds facetious or simply isn't your style, call your therapist or your pastor or the friend you feel best knows you. Go for a long walk in the woods and get it all out.

Here's a healthy panic antidote, especially if you're not good at expressing emotions: Tell your listener that you want to enter a safe, "duty free" zone where you're not taxed for strange, intensely personal or incoherent thinking. Nothing either of you says leaves the room. This is your guiltless chance to express everything on your mind for 15 minutes. But remember to make them stop you when the time is up. Ask your friend to summarize and interpret the salient points without interrupting for at least five minutes. Feedback is a great panic antidote, and giving this forum strict parameters helps you get a handle on it.

Although panic makes you feel like you're losing control of your mind, it's a natural and conditioned response. Your mind is trying to get out of your body, and who can blame it?

Reassure your mind that you're going to take positive action for the good of your body. That you're going to make good decisions about your future. You can do it.

Reaction: Procrastination

If you're feeling fine physically, you may be tempted to say you'll deal with HBV next month or next year, even if your doctor has carefully explained this virus and its consequences to you. This is simply another form of denial. It's also perhaps the most common reaction, since we naturally want to delay unpleasant circumstances as long as possible. We may have the best intentions for getting around to adapting our diet and lifestyle, but everything can wait just a little longer, can't it? Is one more margarita really going to make a difference?

Unfortunately, procrastination is a belief that time is not our master. But days can conveniently slide into months and months into years. And that just won't cut it in the world of HBV. You need to try to get your viral load down as soon as possible to decrease the risk of developing serious progressive liver disease.

Reaction: Obsession

The opposite of procrastination and denial is obsession. There is a fine line between being proactive about your health and being totally obsessive about HBV. Unfortunately there are those of us who actually seem to enjoy talking about their condition, using the disease for attention. Although I believe it is essential to learn as much as you can about HBV, I also believe that it should not be a substitute for an actual life.

An imaginary alarm goes off in my head if I speak for more than five minutes about HBV and its symptoms with someone who is curious about my condition or the disease. I usually talk about how important it is to get tested and vaccinated and how I'm feeling overall, then I attempt to change the subject. I'd much rather talk about how quickly my tomatoes are growing or how talented my nieces and nephews are. I want people to know that HBV is important to me, but it is not my only focus. There is a huge difference between being well informed and being sucked in. You don't want people to think you have nothing else on your mind; otherwise you become a total HBV geek.

HBV doesn't have to seep into your identity. This is how my friend and fellow hepatitis author Hedy Weinberg aptly put it in a recent hepatitis conference: "I am not my illness. I have a core, a soul, that is not touched by hepatitis."

Reaction: Cyber overload

Being proactive about our own wellbeing while listening to our hearts will take us far even after our diagnosis, if we approach the reality of HBV with determination, conviction, and sensitivity. With technology at our fingertips and search engines at our beck and call, however, we may feel compelled to go overboard. Be aware that doctors will very likely perceive us as know-it-alls (or reckless rookies) if we walk into their offices with folders of printouts from the Web.

Gathering information indiscriminately won't help our doctors or us. A good deal of information is posted on the Web without any research to back it up, so we have to be extra vigilant about the quality and veracity of our data. In the partnership you form with your doctor, try to find a happy medium where the research you gather acts as fodder for questions—not affirmatives.

IN A SENTENCE:

> *There are many common reactions to being diagnosed with HBV, but knowing about a few of the most common will help you gain some perspective about what you're going through today.*

learning

What is Hepatitis?

HEPATITIS WAS first described in ancient Chinese writings. In the West, descriptions of liver disease appear as early as 751 A.D. in letters from Pope Zacharias to the Archbishop of Mainz. There are many accounts of outbreaks over the centuries, particularly in times of war. But serious study of the disease didn't really begin until after World War II, when several million doses of yellow fever vaccine tainted with HBV were administered to the U.S. Army. As a consequence, thousands of soldiers became infected, and since that historical tragedy, hepatitis is no longer perceived as a disease specific to unsanitary environments.

Hepatitis is the broad term we use to describe a variety of causes of inflammation of the liver. It is important to remember that viruses aren't the only cause of liver inflammation. Medications, some herbs, alcohol, toxins, chemicals, injuries, obesity, and other diseases can also cause hepatitis.

Another less common kind of hepatitis is caused by an autoimmune disorder, which occurs when our body gets confused and starts attacking our livers. As you can imagine, a combination of any of these causes will make treatment decisions and various symptoms even more complicated. Surprisingly, it wasn't until the 1940s that the two routes of infection—food-borne and blood-borne—were identified and distinguished.

"Infectious hepatitis" is just a way to say that we get it by drinking infected water or eating infected food. Hepatitis A (HAV) is a food-borne virus.

"Serum hepatitis" is transmitted via contact with infected blood. Hepatitis B virus (HBV) and hepatitis C (HCV) are examples of serum hepatitis. Hepatitis C is not as contagious as hepatitis B and is usually associated with blood transfusions or intravenous injections or needle sticks. Transmission of HCV via bodily fluids is uncommon but possible. "Non-A, Non-B" is actually sometimes still used to describe HCV, but the usage is outdated.

Hepatitis D (HDV, or Delta hepatitis) is blood-borne, and infects only those who have HBV, though not all of those with HBV are co-infected with HDV. The presence of HDV may cause your hepatitis B to result in more serious damage to your liver. Hepatitis E (HEV), like hepatitis A, is transmitted via the fecal-oral route.

A total of six types of the hepatitis virus have been identified: A, B, C, D, E and G. Why did they skip F? In the early 1990s something creatively called *Non A-B-C-D-E* was thought to have been identified in Japan, and so the position in the nomenclature was reserved. Further studies, however, failed to corroborate the evidence, and so we have what amounts to a placeholder.

What about hepatitis B?

Dr. Baruch Blumberg discovered the hepatitis B virus in 1965. At the time, Dr. Blumberg was investigating genetic differences between races and their susceptibility to disease by studying how **antibodies** react against antigens. While he was collecting and studying blood samples from indigenous populations around the world, Blumberg noticed that antibodies in two patients receiving blood from an Australian aborigine reacted against an antigen. In 1966 he started collaborating with Alfred Prince, a virologist at the New York Blood Center. Prince was interested in transfusion hepatitis and believed that Blumberg's "Australian antigen" was linked to HBV.

In 1967 it was confirmed that a marker for HBV had been discovered, meaning that blood could be tested, epidemiology could be traced, and a vaccine could be developed. Amazingly, within only two years, Blumberg and Irving Millman invented the HBV vaccine. Dr. Blumberg was awarded the Nobel Prize in 1976; his is one of the great medical discoveries of the twentieth century.

Since the early 1970s blood banks have required donor blood to be tested for the surface antigen. Many years later, the virus was finally observed under an electron microscope and the first samples were grown in a test tube in 1986. Each of the six known hepatitis viruses is unique, though all but hepatitis G cause inflammation of the liver.

Hepatitis B is the most common viral infection on earth. It is a **DNA** (deoxyribonucleic acid) virus, a member of the so-called hepadna family of viruses. It has a limited host range, which means that it infects only humans and chimpanzees. Other mammals such as the North American woodchuck and beechey ground squirrels have their own personalized versions of hepadnaviruses. The World Health Organization (WHO) considers HBV to be the most serious type of viral hepatitis. Although it's not much help to those of us already infected by the virus, it is the only form of chronic hepatitis to offer a preventative vaccine. Getting the hepatitis B vaccine can prevent even HDV, as it relies on HBV to survive.

What is a virus?

So what exactly is a virus? It's a tough question to answer. Although a virus mimics a living creature, it is not alive in the way that other organisms are. Nor is a virus inert. A virus is a tiny sycophant or parasite which attaches itself to an unsuspecting living cell. The hepatitis B virus penetrates a liver cell much like a spermatozoid penetrates an egg. Once HBV enters the liver cell, it intuitively heads for the nucleus, where it sets up its operation and releases its contents of DNA and polymerase (chains of **amino acids**) into its surroundings. The sole function of HBV is to reproduce and invade other living cells.

Like a guest who won't ever leave, the virus makes itself at home, raids the refrigerator of the cell's nucleus, and exploits the cell's components and enzymes. Then the crafty polymerases actually convince the liver cell, a Good Samaritan in any other context, to make components of HBV DNA from **RNA** (ribonucleic acid, an essential building block for the replication of the virus), at which point the well-intentioned cell starts to create copies of the hepatitis B virus. In essence, the virus forces our liver cells to manufacture components that will eventually become spare parts for other hepatitis B viruses. A morbid codependence between the cell and the virus ensues.

Copies of the virus created by this partnership are then released from the liver cell into the bloodstream, killing off the host cell and infecting other healthy liver cells. The whole process can take as little as a few hours, but must happen many times over for significant damage to occur.

Viruses are often confused with bacteria since they both cause a multitude of illnesses. Yet viruses are so small that they can, at times, infect bacteria just as bacteria and viruses infect humans. You may be wondering why antibiotics are useless against HBV. Since HBV lives *inside* the liver cells, the antibiotic would have to kill the liver cells to kill the virus, causing further damage to the liver.

The immune system

Our immune system is also well-intentioned, so much so that it tries to get rid of the hepatitis B virus by destroying those cells that carry it. Unfortunately, in this manner, two diametrically opposed objectives meld as the immune system and the virus both use the same strategy: kill the host cell. The virus wants to kill cells for fun and profit, while the other kills cells for survival. That's how hepatitis leads to liver scarring.

The immune system, composed of cells, molecules, and organs, is committed to protecting the body against threats like bacteria, viruses, and fungi. Like the liver, the immune system also carries out its many tasks in a silent and highly effective manner. Every day we inhale or ingest thousands of bacteria and germs. As a consequence, our health depends on the immune system's ability to organize itself: not only does it have to identify the infiltrators, it also has to search out and destroy them.

A few diseases are actually caused by the malfunctioning of our immune system. Allergies, for example, are the result of the immune system's overreaction to foods or stimuli, while diabetes is caused by the immune system's attack on the cells of the pancreas. Another example of this is rheumatoid arthritis, caused by the immune system's mistaken assault on the joints. The immune system's unwarranted attack on the liver is called **autoimmune hepatitis.**

Often people with HBV ask whether is it wise to boost your immune system if you are diagnosed with this particular virus. They are worried that a stronger immune system means more or faster liver cell death and scarring. However, the immune system also produces antibodies, and we need all the antibodies we can get.

IN A SENTENCE:

> HBV, which is the most common form of viral hepatitis, can cause liver inflammation and scarring because some people do not have antibodies to fight the virus.

living

Who Should I Tell?

DISCLOSING INFORMATION about your medical condition is a strictly personal decision. However, once this information is disclosed, it becomes an interpersonal matter. Thus, you must prepare yourself to manage for worst-case (i.e., insensitive and/or ignorant) reactions of those you tell.

Most often friends and acquaintances will be understanding, curious, and gently concerned about your health. On the other end of the spectrum, you may face someone who won't let you kiss them on the cheek or won't let you "trouble yourself" about bringing a dish to the potluck dinner.

How should I tell them?

As a general rule, I find that people tend to match their reaction to the way in which we tell them. If our energy is negative or we appear nervous or upset, most likely they will take their cue from us. By being calm and comfortable, our listeners will be more likely to engage in a discussion about what hepatitis is and how it affects us. Keep it light. This helps foster a healing and healthy dialogue that will continue over time.

You will, most likely, be surprised by empathetic responses like "oh, my cousin has that" or "my aunt had hepatitis" or "I had hepatitis in college, but I can't remember which one." Although not exactly reassuring, it does emphasize that you are not alone.

Telling your partner is tough

Disclosure about your condition is an intensely personal decision. It's not for everyone. And you get better at revealing personal information with time.

This is how Ed Mahoney deals with it: "I have a simple rule when I meet new people. Unless you plan on sleeping with them, it is none of their business. Maybe down the road as you become closer to these people and they know you more fully it might be prudent to let them become aware of your situation. You may need the support of many different people, beyond your family. It is comforting to be able to discuss an aspect of the disease, how I am feeling, test results, etc., with a person close to me. If that is not true in your case then they were never friends to begin with."

But what if you *are* sleeping with this person? There are two main hurdles: medical and emotional. Make sure you and your partner can distinguish between the two. If your partner has not yet been tested, you need to encourage him or her to be tested for HBV. The **incubation period** (the period between initial contact with the virus and the first appearance of markers) varies from 1 to 5 months (typically between 2–3 months), so if the infection is recent it will not be immediately apparent. If the infection was recent, however, and your partner never received the vaccine, he or she should receive hepatitis B immune globulin (HBiG) within 14 days of the initial exposure, and then start the vaccine series.

Giving your partner news that you may have a serious chronic condition is difficult enough. Telling your partner that he or she may also have HBV could be one of the most difficult things you've ever had to face. Waiting for those test results is agonizing.

You probably don't know who gave this to whom, and it really doesn't matter right now anyway. Try not to place blame. Once you have gotten past initial testing, you may feel the need to work on building a new platform of understanding between you and your loved one. It is important to realize that there has been a subtle shift in the vision you have of your future and the dynamic may be changed. This new dynamic will need attention and consideration from both of you. Although the bond you have with your partner doesn't have to be radically different than what you have built together in the past, admitting that there is work to do as a couple to adapt to HBV is healthy and wise.

When issues arise, develop and encourage the reflex of saying, "Can we talk about this now?" or "Time out, let's regroup." HBV can sometimes be an opportunity to solidify and strengthen your existing relationship. You can be a valuable source of information about hepatitis B for your partner and debunk some of its myths in the process. Discussing your relationship in light of the virus can, ideally, bring you and your partner closer together.

Relationship problems aren't always HBV's fault

But of course the world isn't always ideal. Sometimes couples or families can lose perspective in light of HBV. We resort to overgeneralization, looking for easy answers to difficult issues. HBV often becomes a scapegoat for unrelated or preexisting problems.

If your relationship is already going through a tough period, news of HBV can be the final blow. Preexisting anger and resentment will likely be exacerbated by your diagnosis. Seek professional counseling. And if that doesn't seem like a possibility, don't blame HBV or yourself for the breakup—the bad seeds were probably already sown. Let go.

Some people tell everyone

Some people feel the need to tell everyone they know about HBV, and are very upfront and comfortable about it.

I suppose I would fall into that category, with some limits. I almost never offer the information in an unsolicited way. If I imagine that I might have ongoing contact with a person, I prefer for them to form a mental image of me as a healthy, dynamic, and positive person. This can take minutes or it can take months, but I find that it is worth waiting. However, if someone asks me why I'm not drinking my champagne after a toast or eating the homemade ice cream they've delivered to my front door, I initially tell them I have liver problems and have to watch my diet carefully. If they seem particularly interested, understanding, or knowledgeable, I'll tell them that I have HBV. Limiting yourself to telling people that you have a liver problem is a good way to ease into and become accustomed to disclosure. And it's also a good way to ease others into the news of your disease.

In short, if it's relevant to our conversation or if it allows someone to understand me better and, most importantly, if I feel comfortable with this person, I mention it.

There will probably be a wide variety of reactions

It's amazing how differently people react to your news about HBV. Some look pained and scared. Others, already informed and experienced in the subject, ask pertinent, directed questions. There are interesting types who pretend not to have heard what you've said or gloss over it, immediately finding a way to pass on to another subject. Still others offer you a vodka tonic after you tell them, as if nothing has registered.

Alcohol makes it difficult to keep your secret

As mentioned before, you may find yourself having to disclose some kind of personal information, particularly when alcohol is served because many social situations involve alcohol consumption. There are a number of ways you can avoid disclosure, though you may have to tailor your response to the situation at hand. Here are a few lines to give you ideas when you're stuck in a difficult social situation:

○ I'm on a medication and can't mix the two.
    However, if you're not on a medication and don't like lying, this may not be a good option. If you are on a medication this still may not be a good option, as people may not respect your privacy and ask you what medication you're taking.
○ I'm trying to lose weight.
    This line may work at a baby shower, but it probably isn't going to work at a bar.
○ I'm taking a break from alcohol.
    Follow up saying that since you've stopped drinking you feel so much better and have much more energy.
○ I'm getting too old to drink.
    This line works whether you're 21 or 81.
○ I'm trying to be healthier. So far it's working really well.
    Guaranteed to work: no one will have any smart-alecky things to say to this unless you go on to order a cheeseburger with fries and a chocolate malt.

Some people assume that if you're not drinking then you must be in recovery for alcohol addiction. This has happened to me many times. It may bother you that people simply assume that you have an alcohol addiction. Now I don't really care one way or another. If this is an issue for you, use the camouflage technique: nonalcoholic beer in a glass, seltzer, or cranberry juice with a wedge of lime.

Food, like alcohol, may also invite opportunities to tell people about your HBV. If I'm invited to someone's home, I have the choice to keep quiet and confront the possibility of not finding anything I can eat, or I could tell my host that I have a low-fat diet and need something easy to digest. If I remember, sometimes I'll eat something at home before I go so I don't feel so tempted. I'll admit that most of the time I just eat small portions of things I shouldn't, and make up for it the next day by drinking plenty of water or herbal tea and sticking to my diet. Small portions are the key here.

Telling colleagues is your call

If you haven't had any HBV symptoms and treatment isn't affecting your job performance, there's probably no need to risk disclosing your condition. There's no reason your employer needs to know about your HBV, and you have every right to keep it to yourself. You may fear that disclosing your condition will jeopardize your future with the company.

A common fear of employers, especially in smaller companies, is that their insurer may raise rates when it finds out about your chronic condition. As solid as its policies appear to be, your company may assume that since you have HBV you will probably be taking a lot of sick days or will not be performing at full capacity. Perception of you could change among your colleagues. There are many issues to juggle.

However, if your symptoms *do* affect your job performance and your company *doesn't* know you have a chronic condition, you could be fired with no legal recourse. The **Americans with Disabilities Act (ADA)** provides legal protection only if the company has more than 15 employees and is aware of your disability. Even though it's illegal to discriminate against people with diseases like HBV, we'd be naive to believe that there aren't situations where employers invent excuses to get rid of colleagues, or decide to make it difficult for employees to want to stay in their positions. You'll have to play it by ear.

In my case, I decided to tell my boss within the first few weeks of starting my job. I had to. I had been so stressed by the change in jobs that I felt as though I was about to have a flare-up of my symptoms. I looked dragged out. So I knocked on my boss's door. I will never forget the experience. Before I had even finished my little monologue about being chronic, my boss picked up the phone and called his benefits administrator. He asked about his company's short- and long-term disability benefits and immediately gave an order to increase coverage. I had to leave the room in search of Kleenex. It was a beautiful and unexpected gesture of solidarity and understanding.

Deciding whether to switch jobs is also stressful when you have a chronic, preexisting condition. On an emotional level, I prefer stability and low or no stress, and the prospect of transition seems harder to tolerate with my present energy allotment. On a strictly legal level, if you interrupt your benefits in the United States for less than two months, your HBV will not be considered as a preexisting condition. See Month 6 for a discussion about insurance and other work issues.

Telling your children may not be as important as protecting them

It may not be necessary to tell young children about your HBV. But it is critical that you keep razors, manicure tools, toothbrushes, and anything else that might have traces of your blood or bodily fluids out of reach of your children.

Some people shield their children entirely from the news. Iris is one of them, but with reservations: "I don't want my daughter to worry about losing me. I feel bad about hiding it, because it takes me away from closeness that comes with sharing important experiences and feelings, and I want to set an example of not dwelling on it and giving in to it. I want to set an example for facing adversity and not being in denial. But how can I do both?"

Telling the school is not child's play

Legally speaking, you do not have to inform the school of your or your child's HBV. You may be interested to learn that the Center for Disease Control doesn't even advocate that parents of children with HBV inform day cares or schools of their children's status.

A student with hepatitis B isn't a threat to other students or teachers under normal conditions. Hepatitis B is not transmitted through feces, urine, or stool traces in food. In addition, many states now require *immunization* against HBV for students. However, biting or being bitten, scratching hard enough to draw blood, or severe cuts will require universal precautions. If you do not want to disclose your child's condition, you may want to call the school and ask if teachers have been informed about proper universal precautions in these instances.

If you do decide to tell the school, it is important to inform the school that no one save for the officials of the school should be told about the student's condition. You do not want other parents to be informed about your child's condition. Fortunately, there are laws that protect the confidentiality of your private health and educational information. The Family Educational Rights and Privacy Act of 1974 mandates that any institution receiving federal funds be prohibited from divulging student records to any one other than school officials. The Americans with Disabilities Act also protects student medical records. Ironically, mandatory HBV vaccination often forces parents to disclose, since their children do not have the HBV vaccine on their immunization records. Some parents have chosen to simply and effectively avoid this issue by having their HBV-infected children immunized with the HBV vaccine.

Liz chose to tell everyone about her daughter's status: "We chose to tell everyone who needs to know and some that didn't, even though cautioned against it. Overall, it has been met exceptionally well, other than by the local health department nurse and the infectious disease specialist in Miami who had the nerve to ask me why I would bring her here in the first place if we knew she had hepatitis B. Boy did she tick me off!"

Melinda's experience with telling her son's college was also fairly positive: "We have two sons with hepatitis B in college. We didn't see the need to say anything when the older one started college. Wait, I'll take that back. The nurses at the clinic were told because he got bloodwork done there. His close friends at school know he has hepatitis because he did **Interferon** at school, felt like crud, and they all helped out. Did his roommates and friends get the vaccine? No. But fortunately universal precautions are automatic with my sons."

IN A SENTENCE:

> *It's not always easy to know who to tell about your HBV or how to tell them, but there are methods to help you do it in a sensitive and effective way.*

learning

Transmission Modes, Antigens, and Antibodies

Transmission modes

IN ORDER for HBV infection to occur, there must be a source, a transmission mode, and a susceptible host. The source is the person who already has the virus, and anyone who has not been previously infected or immunized is the host, or susceptible to HBV. Hepatitis B is transmitted through direct blood-to-blood or bodily fluid-to-blood contact. As mentioned before, you don't need to do anything special to get it—you get hepatitis B by doing what normal humans do. Although most people with HBV seem not to want to dwell on where they got the virus, here is a list of known risk factors for hepatitis B exposure and potential sources of infection.

In adults:

- Having unprotected sex
- Receiving a blood transfusion or blood product (**platelets**, plasma)
- Sticking yourself with an infected sharp (needle, IV, surgical instrument) if you are a healthcare worker or caregiver

- Snorting drugs with a shared "straw"
- Injecting drugs (legal or illegal) with a shared needle
- Having a manicure/pedicure
- Getting shaved in a barber shop or having a hair cut with infected clippers/scissors
- Getting a tattoo
- Body piercing
- Biting or being bitten by another human being and breaking the skin
- Being born to a HBV positive biological mother
- Living with someone who has HBV, even in the absence of intimate contact
- Having dental work, particularly when blood is involved
- Receiving medical/dental care in a country that reuses its supplies
- Sharing a tooth brush, razor, or other personal grooming supplies
- Working in or being incarcerated in a prison

In children:

- Being born to a mother with HBV
- As a young child, from infected mother, other children or household contacts

Only one occurrence of any the above is sufficient for you to be infected. HBV doesn't care if you are gay or straight, young or old, rich or poor, and it only takes one sex partner or one tattoo to be infected.

The Virology of HBV: Antigens and antibodies

When you are infected with HBV, you are infected with antigens, and in the HBV spaghetti western, antigens wear black and antibodies wear white. The study of these viruses and the markers that identify them is called virology.

What is an antigen? What is an antibody?

Antigens are **protein** molecules and can be thought of as spare parts of viruses that are attached to the surface of invading cells; these molecules elicit an immune response because the body perceives them to be a threat.

Antibodies are also protein molecules, however they are produced as a reaction by **lymphocytes**, a type of white blood cell that fight antigens.

Antibodies actually adapt their molecular structure to lock into the structure of an antigen so that the interlocking proteins can be disposed of by the immune system, which recognizes the antibody's structure. There are five major classifications of antibodies, which you can always recognize by the suffix -Ig, short for **immunoglobulin**.

In a nutshell, antigens are bad and antibodies are good. Generally speaking, if you have two or more HBV antigens present in your blood, that's not a good sign. The presence of two or more HBV antibodies in your blood is good.

Sometime it's hard to keep medical terms straight; it may help to think that when there are millions of antigens and antibodies in our systems, our bodies get confused and struggle to tell the difference between the good guys and the bad guys. The body thinks it has plenty of antibodies running around so it doesn't make any more; that's why our illness is chronic. In clinical shorthand, Ag identifies antigens, while antibodies are shortened to Ab.

Antigens and antibodies are made up of various components in the bloodstream and can be detected by tests. There are three antigen-antibody systems associated with HBV infection. These are the foundation for HBV testing, what your doctor calls hepatitis serology. You've already seen the following names on your test results.

Surface antigen and antibody—HBsAg and HBsAg. Nickname: Surface or S. The surface antigen is the earliest indicator of acute HBV infection, but does not distinguish between acute and chronic infection. You will sometimes see HBsAg referred to as anti-HBs, but to avoid confusion it is best to only use HBsAg.

Core antigen and antibody—HBcAg and HBcAb (also known as IgM anti-HBc and IgG anti-HBc) Nickname: Core or C. It is nicknamed "core" because it is found at the core of the virus. It is hard to test for and is not available for routine use. However, antibody to the core antigen is usually helpful to distinguish between acute and chronic infection. Sometimes the interpretation of the core antibody test wholly depends on the surface antigen and antibody results. The presence of core antibody means that additional blood tests and medical follow-up are necessary.

E antigen and antibody—HBeAg and HBeAb. Nickname: "e." The e antigen is very often present in people who have an acute HBV infection and in some people with chronic infection, and signifies that the virus is actively and rapidly reproducing in your blood. It is the most dependable and direct measure of infectivity. As mentioned before, people with both HBsAg and HBeAg are usually quite infectious. People who are e negative or who have e antibodies are usually less infectious. People who have antibodies to the e antigen can still be chronic but they usually have an inactive infection (inactive carrier state).

I'm not going to give you a pop quiz about these components, and I don't expect this language to sink in right away. If you don't remember anything else, remember that:

- ○ HB = Hepatitis B
- ○ Ag = Antigen
- ○ Ab = Antibody
- ○ Antigens = Bad
- ○ Antibodies = Good
- ○ Two or more antibodies is a good thing
- ○ Two or more antigens is not a good thing.

Chronic infection is diagnosed when we maintain a positive blood test for the surface antigen HBsAg for six or more months. Chronic HBV people may have normal liver function tests or they can have abnormal ALT/AST levels and various degrees of underlying liver damage. Each year, only one to two percent of these individuals will spontaneously lose the hepatitis B virus and convert from HBsAg to HBsAb positive. Other nonchronic people develop the antibody to HBsAg either after an acute case of HBV or after being vaccinated. Often doctors will test blood for anti-HBs to find out about previous infections or to determine whether vaccination is really necessary. This antibody protects a person from any future HBV infection.

It is even possible that both the surface antigen and antibody coexist in the body, and if this is true for a person, he or she is treated just like those who only have the surface antigen.

The e antigen

You will be hearing the terms *e negative* or *e antigen positive* when speaking to your doctor or fellow HBV friends. What is the e antigen and why is it so important? Discovered in 1973, the e antigen is a peptide (linked amino acids) and partner in crime of HBV. It acts as a supercharger, causing us to be particularly infectious when we carry it in our bloodstream.

Unfortunately, it also increases the likelihood that HBV will lead to liver damage. A protein, it acts like a protective coating on the virus and seems to protect the infected liver cell from our immune system's attack. This allows the cell to continue harboring the spare parts so necessary for viral replication and inhibits the immune system's response. The presence of the e antigen, therefore, means that HBV is actively replicating in your body.

The first goal of treatment for HBV is to **seroconvert**, or lose, the e antigen, and then possibly develop antibodies against it. One to three percent will spontaneously seroconvert annually without undergoing treatment. If you don't seroconvert spontaneously and don't respond to treatment, there is still a chance that you can do so later. Unfortunately, sometimes we lose the e antigen and become less infectious because the virus seems to lose interest in us only after it has taken its toll on our livers. Other times we can regain the e antigen after months or years of remission. As mentioned before, we call this flip-flopping, a fairly common and annoying occurrence. This is yet another reason we must keep getting tested every few months. HBV is the perfect, unpredictable parasite.

It takes about 1 to 6 months for the hepatitis B virus to incubate in the human body, but only a few weeks for the antigens to be detectable in lab tests. In any case, you will be asked to return for tests every three or four months, even if you eventually lose the e antigen.

HBV Markers

Your blood test results will identify the positive or negative presence of antigens or antibodies in your bloodstream via **markers**.

Here is a table of HBV markers—although it looks daunting, you can try using it to check or doublecheck your own HBV test results:

Antigens and Antibodies						
What do my test results mean?						
HBsAg (S Antigen)	HBeAg (E-Antigen)	Anti-HBe (E-Antibody)	Anti-HBcIgm	Anti-HBcIgG	Anti-HBs	Interpretation
–	–	–	–	–	–	Susceptible to HBV infection
–	–	–	–	+	+	Immune due to natural infection
+	+	–	–	–	–	Incubation
+	+	–	+	+	–	Acute HBV
+	+	–	–	+	–	Active carrier

Antigens and Antibodies (continued)

HBsAg (S Antigen)	HBeAg (E-Antigen)	Anti-HBe (E-Antibody)	Anti-HBcIgm	Anti-HBcIgG	Anti-HBs	Interpretation
+	−	+/−		+		Inactive carrier
−	−	+	−	+	+	Convalescence Period
−	−	−	−	+	+	Full Recovery
−	−	−	+	+	−	Acute HBV infection with no detectable HBsAg
−	−	−	−	+	−	Recovery with loss of detectable Anti-Hbs
−	−	−	−	−	+	Immunization without infection or recovery from HBV infection with no detectable IgG anti-HBc

What is seroconversion?

Seroconversion literally means that one or more antigens or antibodies has changed from negative to positive or vice versa. Most of the time we use this term to say that we've lost the e antigen and developed the e antibody. E antigen seroconversion is a more precise term for this occurrence. It's definitely a cause for celebration, as it means that the virus is no longer replicating in our blood.

Some of us will further seroconvert by losing the s antigen (HBsAg) and gaining the s antibody (HBsAb). Referred to as s antigen conversion, this event calls for a really big party (with lots of nonalcoholic champagne).

IN A SENTENCE:

Hepatitis B can be quite infectious, and knowing about your antibodies and antigens is essential for gauging how your body copes with the infection.

Finding Others
Like You

ONCE YOU'VE started getting used to the idea of having HBV, you can start connecting with others who understand what you're going through. One of the perks of having HBV is that you have the chance to make new friends from all walks of life and from all over the world.

Start with the Hepatitis B Information and Support Listserv

If you have access to a computer and the Internet at home or at your local library or Internet cafe, you may want to think about joining the Hepatitis B Information and Support Listserv operated by Steve Bingham and Sheree Martin. A listserv is a public arena of e-mail, in which everyone's messages are sent to everyone. They are not posted on the Internet, but if you reply to an e-mail, your message is also sent to everyone on the list.

To subscribe to the Hepatitis B Information and Support Listserve, all you have to do is send a blank e-mail to hepatitis-b-on @mail-list.com and you will instantly plug into a caring network connecting you to hundreds of other people from all over the world. The support group is actually a daily mailing of e-mails about topics of interest to the group. You can also request a digest version that cuts down on the number of e-mails you receive in your inbox or temporarily stop e-mails while you're on vacation.

You can be as visible or invisible as you like on the list. If you feel uncomfortable with coming out to others and choose to remain incognito, you can even be a lurker, which means that you read but don't post questions or comments.

I like Steve and Sheree's group because they have a vast amount of experience with HBV and have access to fresh research, articles, and statistics. They have many other good qualities too: understanding ears, patience, warmth, openness, and a passion for getting to the heart of HBV issues. They are also a lot of fun. I have kept every single one of the support group's e-mails in my inbox (to the chagrin of my hard drive) for fear of losing pertinent information that may be helpful down the line.

There is no substitute for shooting a burning question to the list and getting answers in real-time from fellow list-members and doctors. Even some of the pharmaceutical companies and government agencies monitor the list. The listserv also provides a crosscultural perspective on HBV since its membership is located in dozens of countries worldwide.

Sheree and Steve also keep an archive of topics and articles that you can reference when you like. You can search the archive with a keyword and quickly obtain a list of documents that you can read online, download, or print.

A graduate student named Chari Cohen recently conducted a study on the group, revealing that the HB-L list is a very effective forum for discussing HBV. The study shows that 82 percent of list members feel that they get more valuable information from the list than from their physicians, and 74 percent say that good information is hard to get anywhere else. Fifty-three percent have altered their diet based on what they've learned from the list.

Fortunately, there are a few good-natured researchers, doctors, and other health care professionals who kindly step in when clarification or corrections are needed. It never ceases to amaze me how many levels of knowledge there are regarding HBV, and how we've just scratched the surface.

Internet newsletters and magazines

B-Informed, the free newsletter of the Hepatitis B Foundation (HBF), is a great resource for the latest news in treatment, diet, supplements, research, and resources. You can get a copy online at www.hepb.org or request to be put on their mailing list.

The Immunization Action Coalition (IAC) will automatically send you news about HBV diagnosis and treatment if you subscribe to the *IAC Express*. Their weekly online publication covers a wide range of issues and topics. Some of the information may be a bit technical for newcomers, but you will also receive general news from the Center of Disease Control and recent press releases about hepatitis in general. Send a blank e-mail to www.express@immunize.org.

Check your local chapter of the American Liver Foundation to see if they have their own newsletter. My local Chicago chapter distributes a bimonthly about local events, seminars, and fund-raisers. Local medical professionals are frequent contributors, and most issues contain a directory of liver resources. Call the national hotline 1-800-GO-LIVER or go to www.liverfoundation.org.

Hepatitis Magazine is the only national publication dedicated to people with HBV and HCV. Published bimonthly, it is a good resource guide and provides current, comprehensive information. You can find subscription information and various articles from previous issues at the website: www.hepatitismag.com. They also occasionally organize conferences for people with hepatitis.

You may find it discouraging to see that most sites and publications focus exclusively on HCV. This isn't necessarily a bad thing and certainly isn't, in most cases, intended to be exclusionary. The fact is that HCV behaves quite differently from HBV, so it can be especially confusing to see information about particular treatment strategies and terminology, especially when you've just been diagnosed. Better to keep them separate. You can, however, feel free to raid the HCV sites for information regarding diet, emotional, financial, or legal issues.

Web resources

Your starting point should be the Hepatitis B Foundation's excellent site (see above). The HBF is a voluntary, nonprofit organization dedicated solely to the cause and cure of chronic hepatitis B through research, education, and patient support. You will find a wealth of in-depth information on their site. There are other relevant sites, such as the Hepatitis Neighborhood (www.hepatitisneighborhood.com), a veritable Web community. They often organize online "town halls," where you can ask questions in real-time about various topics. If you choose, you can receive advance notice of these meetings via e-mail. And if you miss the town hall meeting you can find an archive of past meetings and print out the transcripts. There are also real-time chat rooms on selected topics.

Hepatitis Central (http://hepatitis-central.com) offers extensive information about hepatitis, along with a listing of hepatologists in the United States. Much of the information refers to HCV, but you can find good resources on diet and treatment. And another support group geared towards any kind of hepatitis is available at the Yahoo Groups site: http://groups.yahoo.com/group/GIWorld-Hepatitis.

If you're not afraid of technobabble, go to http://dispatch.mail-list.com/archives/hbv_research and search this extraordinary database for articles about treatment, research and a wide range of HBV topics.

The Canadian Liver Foundation (http://www.liver.ca/index.html), the Center for Disease Control (http://www.cdc.gov/ncidod/diseases/hepatitis/hepatitis.htm or phone CDC Hepatitis Hotline, 888-443-7232), the Hepatitis B Information page (http://www.geocities.com/hbvinfo/) and The Hepatitis Information Network (http://www.hepnet.com/) all provide extensive information. And the HIV and Hepatitis site (http://www.hivand-hepatitis.com/) is well-designed and well-organized. It is also very refreshingly well-written. It will be useful to you even if you don't have HIV—just click on the HBV tab to take advantage of their wealth of HBV knowledge.

There are many online chat rooms for people with HCV, but none so far for HBV. No one I've interviewed has ever participated in one. It may be worth trying to create a chat room to see if anyone will join you.

What if I don't have a computer?

It may be time to invest in one. These days, you can find very inexpensive new and used models. If that's not a possibility, see if someone you know will subscribe to the Hepatitis B Information and Support Listserv and let you read the e-mails once a week or print out information that pertains to you. Ask your local librarian for suggestions about how to stay informed and networked. If that's not a possibility either, hopefully your local library will offer free Web access. Use one of the free e-mail providers like Yahoo or Hotmail to set up an e-mail account. Cyber cafes and Internet kiosks are popping up all over, too. And now many cell phones are equipped with Web browsers, so you can check e-mail even if you don't have a computer.

However, until you've become entirely fluent in HBV, be wary of information you get from the Web. Some will be outdated even if it was published last year. Some information will be biased or sponsored by large corporations with specific interests, and some may simply not apply to your specific case. You can also just pick up a phone and dial the Hepatitis B Foundation at (215) 489-4900 and speak immediately to a live person who will help answer your questions or concerns. They'll even call you back if you're on a budget.

Why aren't there local support groups?

It's embarrassing to say that there don't seem to be any existing brick-and-mortar HBV support groups in the United States. You can find hundreds for individuals with hepatitis C. Perhaps *you* should offer to start an HBV group.

IN A SENTENCE:

> *If you have a computer or access to the Web, there are plenty of online resources to help you learn more about HBV and to give you the support and information you need.*

learning

Understanding Your Lab Tests

Liver Function Tests (LFTs)

AS WE learned in the last chapter, there are various tests that measure specific antigens and antibodies in your blood. These are called direct markers, since they directly correlate to what your immune cells are doing (or not doing) in response to the presence of antigens.

Liver function tests, also known as LFTs, are referred to as indirect markers because these blood tests evaluate the condition of your liver in a more indirect way. The term liver function test is a bit of a misnomer since there aren't hard and fast rules regarding these markers, and most of these tests gauge the severity of damage that occurs in the liver rather than actual hepatic functioning. The most common LFTs are ALT and AST, **bilirubin** and **albumin**, and **prothrombin time.**

Liver enzymes

Liver enzymes are actually proteins produced by the liver. These enzymes help facilitate chemical reactions in the body. Elevated levels of enzymes, however, are a red flag. They show that liver cells are rupturing (in a process called **hepatocyte necrosis**) and leaking these proteins into the blood system.

Whether you have chronic or acute hepatitis B, you will be asked to have tests done quite often, depending on your condition and your doctor's recommendation. Having these tests is one of the most important things you can do to protect your health. In the months following your diagnosis you may even be asked to come in for a blood draw every month. After your diagnosis is confirmed, you may drop down to 2–4 times a year.

ALT

ALT is short for alanine **aminotransferase**. Blood test results sometimes list it by its former name, **SGPT** (**serum glutamic-pyruvic transaminase**). You will often hear your doctor or other HBV friends say, "My ALT is normal" or "My enzymes went through the roof." Since ALT is found only in the liver, it is a more specific indicator of liver inflammation than AST.

These enzymes are measured by international units per liter **IU/L**, the most common measurement standard. Although every laboratory has slightly different ranges, normal ALT levels fall roughly within the following ranges:

Adults: 10–40 IU/L,
Children: 5–30 IU/L
Newborns: 1–25 IU/L.

ALT levels may indicate different liver diseases or injuries. Compared to AST, ALT is less sensitive to alcoholic liver disease (see below).

Low ALT levels can be a sign of uremia, malnutrition, or even successful hepatitis treatment, which can lower levels beyond low normal range. In chronic liver disease these enzymes sometimes appear within the normal range despite the presence of cirrhosis. Some medications can increase ALT levels. These may be nonspecific, although in rare cases they can result in severe liver injury. ALT is also highly sensitive to alcohol consumption. Even after one drink, your ALT can rise. ALT can spike if you do intense physical activity.

My ALT has ranged from 20 to 600 over the years, so I've had the opportunity to experience the full spectrum of ALT's effect on my energy levels. Here is a simple real-world experience of ALT and its effect on me. Your ALT levels may vary, but you may find it interesting to compare your notes to mine and gauge how you feel at various ALT levels since they don't always correlate with one's symptoms.

Will's ALT	Will's Energy Level
10 to 50	Feel great!
50 to 80	Feel a bit fatigued by dinnertime. I wake up tired.
80 to 125	Feel mildly fatigued and lethargic at intervals all day.
125 to 200	Feel fatigued all day. Sweating at night and itching. Stomach feels queasy.
200 to 500	Feel very fatigued all day. Need to take naps. Limbs feel heavy. Skin is pale; there are dark circles under my eyes. Liver discomfort.
500 +	Hard to get out of bed. Nightsweats and joint aches, dark urine, and itching. Liver feels swollen. No appetite. (Thankfully, this period lasted only a month, and occurred before I started treatment.)

AST

AST (**aspartate transaminase**) is also known as **serum glutamic-oxaloacetic transaminase**, sometimes listed on test results as SGOT, its former acronym. This enzyme is found in numerous organs in the body along with the liver. It is used to monitor cardiac and hepatic diseases. Like ALT, AST is released into blood circulation following the injury or death of cells. The amount of AST in the blood corresponds to the number of damaged cells and the amount of time that passes between injury to the tissue and the test.

Normal ranges of AST:
    Adults: 10–40 UL
    6 days old to 18-year-olds: 10–40 U/L
    0-5 days old: 35–140 U/L

In addition to being an indicator of acute or chronic hepatitis, high AST levels can also be a sign of active cirrhosis, infectious mononucleosis, cancer, alcoholic hepatitis, Reye's syndrome, progressive muscular dystrophy, pulmonary emboli, gangrene, mushroom poisoning, congestive heart failure, exhaustion, and heat stroke, among other diseases. Elevations up to 8 times the normal level may be nonspecific and may be seen in other disorders that are not liver-related. However the highest elevations occur with massive liver damage. Although quite rare, values can go up as high as 10,000 to 15,000 IU in persons with viral hepatitis who make uneventful recoveries.

As with ALT, some medications can increase AST levels: acetaminophen, anesthetic agents, anticonvulsants, antifungals, beta-blockers (blood pressure medications), diuretics, oral contraceptives, and tricyclic antidepressants, to name a few of the more common medications.

Some medications can falsely *lower* the AST level, among which but not limited to are: **milk thistle** (silymarin), acetaminophen, cyclosporine, ketoprofen, metronidazole, prednisone, ursodiol, and vitamin C (and possibly other **antioxidants**).

The higher the AST to ALT ratio, the more likely that alcohol consumption is playing a part in hepatocyte necrosis.

Alkaline Phosphatase (ALP)

ALP is used to detect liver, bile, and bone disorders, and is found in your liver, **biliary tract**, bones, and in the placenta. ALP levels can rise due to bone growth, bile obstruction, or liver disease. High levels of ALP are just one of a few possible signs of cirrhosis, but these levels can also be elevated due to healing fractures, arthritis, and biliary obstruction.

Bilirubin

Bilirubin is a bile pigment and is removed from the bloodstream by the liver. Although it is present even in healthy individuals, an overabundance of this pigment causes jaundice. There are actually two forms of bilirubin in the body, direct and indirect (sometimes called conjugated and unconjugated), and measurement of the two together is known as total Bilirubin or T Bili on lab results.

Bilirubin is considered a true indicator of liver function since it gauges the liver's ability to remove, process, and eventually secrete bilirubin into the bile that is eventually excreted from our bodies. Healthy people have almost no bilirubin in their blood.

Total bilirubin should be around or less than one, but a high bilirubin level is not necessarily due only to liver disease. **Hemolysis** (breakdown of red blood cells), obstruction of the bile duct outside the liver due to stones, pancreatitis, or cancer of the bile duct can also cause high bilirubin levels.

It is a good idea to avoid eating yams, carrots, or high-fat meals before this test, as they can affect the reading. Doctors will often ask you to describe the color of your stools to get an idea about how your body is dealing with bile, as light-colored feces are a sign that the body is not efficiently eliminating bilirubin, especially in instances of bile-duct obstruction.

GGT

Gamma Glutamyl transerase is another enzyme present in the kidney, liver, and pancreas. **GGT** is often elevated in persons who take three or more alcoholic drinks, and is a useful marker for alcohol intake and alcohol-induced liver disease. It is also elevated in people taking anticonvulsants like Dilantin or barbituates. When abnormal levels of GGT are present along with alkaline phosphatase, it may be a sign of a biliary problem or obstruction in the bile duct.

GGT doesn't get a whole lot of attention compared to other lab tests as it can be quite nonspecific, and its score must be placed into context with other enzymes.

Serum Albumin

Albumin is a protein that is formed in the liver. Liver disease causes a decrease in albumin, which can lead to **ascites** (fluid in the abdomen) or **edema** (fluid in the legs). If you have low levels of albumin, it is particularly important that you stay properly hydrated, as albumin levels can fluctuate according to variations in the body's hydration.

The normal range is 3.5 to 5.0 gm/dl. (Note: gm/dl = grams per deciliter)

The presence of albumin in the urine can be indicative of kidney disease (which may be due to HBV) or heart disease. Note that albumin should not be confused with albumen, which is the white of an egg.

Prothrombin Time

You've most likely given blood for a Prothrombin test if you've already had your first liver biopsy. Although it is an approximate measure of liver function, high levels could mean the liver is beginning to have trouble functioning. Some drugs, such as blood thinners, can raise your Prothrombin time. Also, by gauging risk from bleeding along with the other tests (such as platelets) that measure your blood's ability to clot, prothrombin helps determine if it is safe to perform a **percunateous biopsy**.

Normal range is approximately 11–14 seconds (3 seconds or less from a healthy control).

You may be tested for Hepatitis D, C, and HIV

If your doctor feels that your hepatitis is particularly active, he will want to know if you also have hepatitis C, D, and/or HIV, as co-infection is not unusual in those who already have HBV. HDV is actually a defective virus that needs HBV to exist. HDV acts as a kind of hepatitis supercharger, potentially damaging your liver more quickly than would HBV alone. In fact, while only 20 percent of those with HBV progress toward cirrhosis, as much as 60 percent of those co-infected with HDV go on to cirrhosis. Co-infection with HDV may also influence your treatment strategy, as those with both strains may not respond well to currently available treatments.

Roughly 10–14 percent of those with HIV and 3–18 percent of those with HCV test positive for HBV antibodies, so it is wise to check for either upon your diagnosis, and it is a good idea to continue practicing safe sex. If you're sexually active, you may want to ask your doctor to run tests for HIV and HCV regularly.

HBV DNA/PCR

HBV can be measured in the blood by different **assays**, or tests. The most sensitive is the **polymerase chain reaction** (**PCR**), a highly sensitive (and expensive) test that can detect extremely small quantities of DNA or RNA. It does so by forcing DNA to amplify or multiply in a tube. This test measures the quantity of HBV DNA in your blood, and is often referred to as your viral load. Once used mainly for research purposes, it is now more frequently used by doctors for special diagnostic purposes.

If you know that your viral load is quite low (under 200,000 copies/ml) you should check to make sure you are being tested via PCR testing and not by what is called a branched chain DNA test. Otherwise you might receive a false negative result for DNA since the branched chain test is not sensitive enough. Those who are currently being treated should also make sure that they're having a PCR done rather than a branched chain.

Ranges vary and are quoted in pg/mL or copies/ml (virions/mL) of blood, depending on whether the lab has done the conversion between pg and copies of virions. It can be very confusing to convert the two since various labs have different equations. In general, the conversion standard is somewhere between 240,000 and 260,000 copies per picogram. Most labs now round off the figure and use 250,000 copies per pg/ml.

Here is a conversion table to help you:

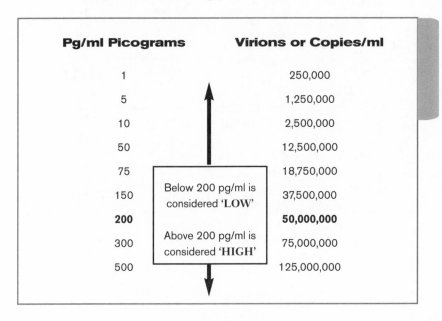

Pg/ml Picograms	Virions or Copies/ml
1	250,000
5	1,250,000
10	2,500,000
50	12,500,000
75	18,750,000
150	37,500,000
200	**50,000,000**
300	75,000,000
500	125,000,000

Below 200 pg/ml is considered 'LOW'

Above 200 pg/ml is considered 'HIGH'

Knowing if your viral load is high or low is important

Viral load is important when deciding on a particular treatment strategy, and it also measures the efficacy of treatment as it progresses. Clinical trials have shown that a HBV DNA load of less than 200 pg/ml is low and has a favorable outcome on treatment. Anything above this value is considered a high viral load. Viral load is typically an accurate barometer of how serious your symptoms will be.

Ultrasounds and CT scans

Ultrasound is an imaging technique that uses high frequency sound waves and their echoes to obtain an image of your internal organs. The technique is similar to the sonar used by submarines.

Having an ultrasound may just become your favorite test because it's painless. It is one more way the doctor can determine how your liver is doing, though it is not nearly as informative as a biopsy. It is usually recommended that you get an ultrasound at **baseline** and on a periodic basis (every 6–12 months) depending on your potential risk for liver cancer (in particular for Asians, those with cirrhosis, or a family history of liver cancer). The ultrasound checks the shape of your liver and makes sure that there are no abnormalities. Although ultrasound is a helpful safeguard against large masses, it cannot tell the difference between malignant (cancerous) and benign (noncancerous) masses, and thus is not a replacement for a biopsy.

You will be asked to fast for 12 hours before the exam, so you may want to schedule an early appointment. The ultrasound will most likely be performed by a radiologist, but there won't be any radiation from the ultrasound. You'll be asked to take your clothes off above your waist and lay down on a table next to the machine. Some warm (if you're lucky) lubricant will be applied to your abdomen by the technician and what looks like a padded mouse will be guided over your liver. You can usually turn your head to watch the dark images of your organs appear on the monitor. I recommend having a look. Often the radiologist will point out your various organs to you: liver, kidneys, spleen, and gallbladder. The entire procedure lasts only about 10 minutes.

Some doctors prefer to use CT (**computerized tomography**) scans, which show a cross section of your abdomen. Other doctors avoid them because they expose you to low doses of radiation. MRIs (magnetic resonance imaging) are a good alternative, but they are very expensive.

You may be asked to undergo an endoscopy

Your specialist may suggest an upper **gastrointestinal endoscopy**, especially if you have cirrhosis. Carried out under light sedation, this procedure entails the use of a fiber-optic tube that is passed down your throat to examine your esophagus and stomach for the presence of **varices**. Varices are distended twisted veins that look like **varicose veins** in legs. They develop in the esophagus and stomach in the presence of cirrhosis, and are one of the more serious consequences of long-term HBV infection. Varices are important to document because they can rupture and cause severe bleeding. It is critical to be aware of this preventable and treatable danger when you have cirrhosis, because it can be fatal if not treated immediately. There will be an in-depth discussion of HBV-related complications in Month 8.

IN A SENTENCE:

Understanding your blood tests can be quite difficult and confusing, but will eventually help you make good decisions about treatment.

DAY 5

living

Get a Specialist

IF YOU have hepatitis B, you need a real pro.

If your primary physician or ob-gyn made the diagnosis, he or she may have already recommended that you make an appointment with a GI (gastrointestinal) doctor or hepatologist (liver specialist). It is a good idea to do a little investigating about doctors in your area, and there are resources listed in the back of this book. Ask the new doctor how much of her practice is dedicated to treating hepatitis B, as it is likely you have been referred to a doctor that concentrates on HCV (hepatitis C) or other liver diseases. Some doctors concentrate mainly on transplantation. Clearly, it doesn't hurt to have a doctor who is particularly passionate about HBV.

If your primary physician does not give you a referral for a hepatologist, it may be helpful to do a little research on your own either on the Internet or in a local phone book. Ask HBV support group members if they know and like a particular hepatologist in your area. Many HBV patients say that they wish they had gone directly to a hepatologist right away, instead of relying on their primary physician or GI doctor.

Hepatologists generally have more experience with HBV

Hepatologists are not required to pass a separate board certification exam in order to receive this distinction; however, they very often have completed a few years of in-depth training in the diagnosis and treatment of liver disease. They are very likely to be more comfortable with and informed about the latest developments in hepatitis, and many of them conduct research studies about these treatments with volunteer patients. They also tend to feel less threatened by or uncomfortable with informed patients and more comfortable with new therapies.

Hepatologists train in a liver unit for an extended period of time, and in all probability attend national conferences on hepatitis. They may be members of the American Liver Foundation and may publish articles about studies conducted in the universities where they work. Finally, hepatologists tend to be more willing to let you try the newest medications for HBV or enroll you in a drug trial or experimental study.

However, it should be said that there are some GI doctors who have enormous experience with HBV. If you choose a GI specialist over a hepatologist, you should make sure that your prospective doctor is one of them. Also, none of the people I interviewed would debate that it is worth your while traveling out of your way for a good hepatologist or GI specialist with proven HBV experience.

Your primary physician still plays an important role

You should continue to rely on your primary physician for ongoing health issues other than those relating directly to your liver. Your primary physician can be enormously helpful in providing support in this phase of your life. Hopefully you'll have built a long-lasting relationship with the doctor, and will want to share news about your liver with him. Once you become accustomed to reading about HBV and talking about your liver with other people who have the virus, you may very likely realize that you have as much (or more) fluency in the disease and its treatment as your primary physician. Sometimes they will shoot dozens of questions at you, trying to get a glimpse into your treatment strategy. At times what they say can even seem naive or outdated. Don't despair—that's why you have a specialist.

How to find the right doctor

Here is a quick rundown of general considerations that are important when looking for any kind of doctor.

Communication—The doctor asks a lot of questions and listens attentively to your answers, doesn't cut you off, refers back to things you said previously, and makes good eye contact. He or she is relaxed yet professional (e.g., shakes your hand or touches your shoulder at the end of the visit). The doctor I saw won me over quite quickly. He sat down very close to me and fixed me in the eye. He also asked me twice if I was sure there wasn't anything else I wanted to talk about. We also found a way to bring laughter into the exam room.

Inquisitiveness—The doctor asks you what your expectations are for the visit, offers to get answers about questions that he/she doesn't know, wonders about your living situation and work dynamic, makes a point of telling you to call back to talk about test results. I love doctors who call me unsolicited after a week to ask me how I'm doing.

Knowledge and Training—Are you more likely to choose a doctor simply because he or she has more credentials? Personally, I want to know how much experience they have with the disease, how many patients they see, how many years they've practiced, where training was received, are they up-to-date on current treatments, do they know about nutrition and alternative therapies? Finally, does the doctor seem to enjoy his work?

Location, location, location—Is the doctor close to your home or office?

Other considerations are of a more administrative nature, but nonetheless important. For example, can you get an appointment in a reasonable time frame? Does the doctor hold late hours at least once a week? Is the doctor available on call after hours? Who is available if the doctor is at a medical conference or on vacation? Is the doctor board-certified? Is the doctor's staff attentive, responsive, friendly, and organized? Is the office clean and orderly? Are the nurses available to answer questions that you might have if the doctor is unavailable?

Try a Web search for the doctor's name before you make an appointment. You might be surprised to find just how many times the doctor's name is mentioned, and hopefully it won't be in lawsuits. I conducted my own Internet investigation on my current doctor, and found information about his training from the American Medical Association. I found an interview in which he spoke about his passion for developing constructive relationships with patients and allowing them to take responsibility for their treatment decisions. Use the Web resources in Month 12 to help you with your search.

Finally, I find it useful to casually interview nurses in the hospital to determine which doctors are most respected by their peers and coworkers. Given that they have firsthand experience with the patient-doctor dynamic, the doctor's public and private selves and treatment decisions over time, nurses have a special perspective on patient satisfaction, thoroughness of follow-up, and organizational skills of the physician. They have almost a paranormal talent for letting you know who's in it for the money and who's in it for love without so much as a word.

Take time to find the right specialist for you

If you have access to the Internet or e-mail, join a hepatitis B online support group. You can ask hundreds of patients for a good referral with just one e-mail. Or try calling your local university medical center and ask for the **Hepatology** department. Ask who on the staff concentrates on hepatitis B. On the Web you can visit the Hepatitis Central site (http://hepatitis-central.com/) for listings in the United States and abroad. You can check out the site of the Hepatitis Foundation International, which lists a toll-free number for a referral in your area. The Hepatitis B Foundation is another excellent resource; for your interest, they also have a listing of hepatologists on their website. Some of the doctors listed on their site can even be contacted by e-mail. The American Association for the Study of Liver Diseases (www.aasld.org) has a directory of hepatologists. You may be disappointed by the American Liver Foundation's site, however, since there is no database of practitioners available. And there are always the Yellow Pages.

Ask a boatload of questions

So you think you have a caring, listening hepatologist lined up. What other questions should you ask? You may want to find out if they do actually treat HBV, inasmuch as certain doctors hold off on current treatment practices in hopes of more effective on-the-horizon treatments. Ask the hepatologist what percentage of their patients have HBV, but don't be surprised if they say only 5–10 percent; remember, there are more than twice as many Americans with hepatitis C than hepatitis B despite the fact that

HBV outnumbers HCV worldwide. Ask the doctor how many liver biopsies the doctor has personally performed over the past year, as one or two biopsies per week would be about the average for an established hepatologist in a larger city. Sometimes, however, hepatologists choose to have radiologists or other doctors in the practice perform biopsies in their place. This is good to know in advance, because you don't want to run into a bait-and-switch when you're already at the hospital. Finally, ask the hepatologist what they think of alternative or Chinese medicine. Even if the doctor doesn't approve of them, it is nonetheless good to know that he or she keeps abreast of new developments on all fronts.

IN A SENTENCE:

Get a hepatologist or GI doctor who specializes in HBV!

learning

Stages and Phases of Hepatitis B

WHICH HBV are you?

When you're first diagnosed, it is hard to know just where you fit in. It seems like there's so much information being thrown at you that you don't know how to determine where you fall on the HBV map. Since HBV manifests itself so differently in different people at different times, it is worthwhile to take a moment to describe the various stages of HBV infection. First we will learn about the phases our immune system goes through when it encounters HBV. Then we will see what stages our livers go through in the years and decades that follow initial infection. Remember: if you were only recently infected with HBV, current treatments may help you avoid more serious liver damage altogether.

Despite all the confusing terminology you might hear, the bottom line is that there are two kinds of HBV: chronic and acute. There are three immune system phases. Then, if our HBV goes unchecked or uncontrolled for many years—even decades—there are various stages of liver disease to contend with: fibrosis, cirrhosis and, possibly, **decompensation** and/or transplantation or liver cancer. Let's get a handle on these various stages.

To start with, here is a diagram showing the natural history of HBV:

Dynamics of HBV Infection

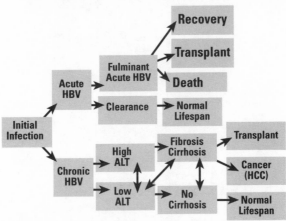

As you can see, there's a fork in the road at every turn, and we can even jump from one path to the next. Again, it is important to remember that it can take many years before you move from one box to the next, if at all.

Immune system phases

HBV does not damage liver cells directly, but creates a dynamic of constant interaction with the immune system and the liver cells, in three consecutive phases.

Immune tolerant phase: In the initial phase your immune system may be tolerant towards HBV and not attack the virus. You may either have normal ALT, be HBeAg positive or negative, or have a high level of HBV DNA. Immune tolerance is common in those who are infected at birth or a very young age. This may occur because a young child's immune system is immature and may not recognize HBV. This phase may last anywhere from one to three decades before entering the immune clearance phase.

Immune clearance phase: Tolerance is followed by active immune-mediated disease, in which the immune system finally realizes that it has to do something about this unwelcome visitor. If clearance of the virus and resolution of disease is going to occur, it will usually happen during this period, which is still within months of initial infection unless, as mentioned above you were infected at a very early age. In the immune clearance stage the e antigen (HBeAg) disappears with the development of the e antibody

(HBeAb). This, in turn, is followed by normalization of liver enzymes in most people.

In some cases, however, seroconversion may cause decompensation of liver disease (see Month 8). HBV core and precore mutations are variations of the HBV virus and can occur during the course of infection, yet their full significance is not fully understood. It is thought that they may alter host response to antiviral therapy (see Month 4 for a more thorough discussion of mutant HBV).

Thus, the frequency, severity, duration, and the extent of acute flares during this phase determines the progress of liver disease and clearance of HBV.

Viral replication and/or integration phase (residual phase): Finally, transition to a phase of reduced viral replication occurs. We say reduced, but that doesn't mean that your viral load won't be quite as high. Some use the term smoldering hepatitis to describe this phase. At some stage during the course of chronic hepatitis B, the HBV genome (the molecular structure of the virus) integrates into our **hepatocyte** (liver cell) DNA, though we don't exactly know when this happens and how this affects subsequent disease progression. The dynamics of viral replication and/or integration is different and as individual as a fingerprint.

Chronic HBV infection behaves differently in Caucasians and Asians

Since many Asians are infected in early childhood or at birth, they may have a longer immune tolerance phase followed by frequent flares in the immune clearance stage. If you are Asian you may be more prone to serious liver damage because each flare results in an attack on the liver. Over time these accumulated attacks can cause progressive, serious liver scarring. But it is important to remember that sometimes a flare is a precursor to HBeAg seroconversion to HBeAb. Caucasians generally tend to be infected later in life, so if they develop the e antibody without detectable HBV DNA they have a lower risk of cirrhosis and liver cancer. This risks being over-generalized (not all Asians are infected at birth; not all Caucasians are infected as adults), but is nonetheless good to be informed about.

Acute hepatitis is more common than chronic hepatitis

Acute hepatitis B takes anywhere from 4 weeks to 32 weeks after exposure to show itself either by signs and symptoms or in blood work. However, for a period not lasting longer than 6 months, the virus is actively replicating and damaging liver cells, which can lead to elevated enzyme levels. Most people with acute HBV never know they've had it and get over it without any symptoms whatsoever. The virus tends to keep us from getting too sick so we can go merrily on our way, infecting others. Symptoms that do appear may be similar to other diseases or discomforts: depression, the common flu, loss of appetite, nausea, bloating and/or irritable bowel, itching, or sensitivity to smells. Some smokers may notice that they no longer like the taste of their brand or can't tolerate smoke at all. The following chart demonstrates what happens to your markers when you are acute:

Markers in Acute Hepatitis B

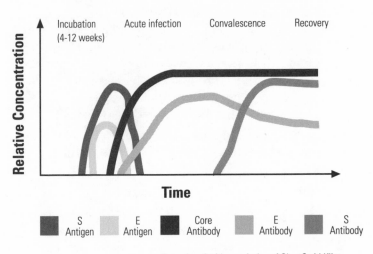

Reproduced with permission of GlaxoSmithKline

Alarm and shock, however, may characterize acute HBV in the presence of more apparent symptoms like jaundice or swelling of the liver. It is also possible to experience symptoms that are due to reservoirs of HBV outside of the liver, such as joint aches, kidney problems, dermatitis, or neuropathy. These are called extra-hepatic manifestations of HBV. Extra-hepatic HBV can also occur in those who are chronic.

People with acute HBV have a good chance (90 percent) of clearing the virus completely, but they should also be on the lookout for early warning signs of fulminant hepatitis (0.1 to 1 percent) such as altered mental state or **encephalopathy**. If you have chronic HBV and are experiencing an acute flare, you have a good chance of responding to Interferon treatment and will probably lose the e antigen.

Decades of chronic active hepatitis lead to various levels of scarring

Chronic hepatitis is a different bird—what your hepatologist calls a distinct clinical entity. It is characterized by 6 months or more of:

○ Clinical symptoms or liver disease or total absence of symptoms
○ Elevated liver enzymes (not caused by obesity, alcohol abuse, fatty liver, or drugs)
○ Evidence of chronic disease on ultrasound/CT scan/MRI or abnormal results seen in your liver tissue after liver biopsy
○ Presence of HbeAg unless you are infected with an HBV variant like the **precore mutant**.

Unfortunately, this stage is also very often characterized by blissful ignorance, as most of us do not manifest signs or symptoms of the disease in the initial stage. The following graph clearly illustrates that there is no variation of markers over time:

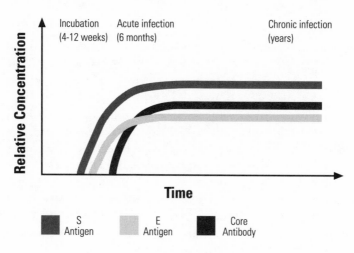

Markers in Chronic Active Hepatitis B

Reproduced with permission of GlaxoSmithKline

In these people HBsAg remains positive and HBsAb does not develop, and they may have ongoing virus replication as seen by elevated liver enzymes and inflammation on their tissue samples. The actively replicating virus continuously damages the liver cells, causing elevated enzyme levels. These people have a good chance of responding to Interferon treatment and have small chance of spontaneously losing the e antigen or even clearing the virus completely (see next graph).

Those with active infection either experience high or low replication of the virus in their system. Those with high replication may experience more of the classic symptoms of HBV infection: fatigue, aches in the joints, itching. This is the stage of chronic hepatitis with activity, also known as chronic active or aggressive hepatitis.

HBV simmers but doesn't boil over

This stage has a few aliases: silent carrier, or healthy carrier, or simply persistent hepatitis. In short, it is a smoldering stage of hepatitis, in which HBV simmers but doesn't boil over. In this common stage, people have been HBsAg positive for more than six months with normal or near normal enzymes and normal or minimally abnormal biopsies. They may have a low or even no viral load. The infection is almost entirely **asymptomatic**. They have only a 1 percent chance of spontaneously seroconverting, or losing the e antigen. Many silent carriers have had HBV since birth.

Hepatitis B chronic carrier with e antigen seroconversion

The following chart shows the loss of the e antigen and development of the e antibody. This is a positive development, and it means that your HBV is no longer actively replicating. It also means that you are no longer highly contagious.

I've heard the term burnt out hepatitis B used to describe those of us who have no detectable virus with positive hepatitis B surface antigens, and this indicates that we have the virus in the nucleus of our liver cells but don't have virus in our blood any longer. HBV is not actively causing liver inflammation or damage, but that doesn't mean it can't flare up again.

These people tend not to respond well to Interferon, because as Steve Bingham poetically puts it, "the gophers have to stick their heads out before

Markers in Chronic Hepatitis B with E-antigen Seroconversion

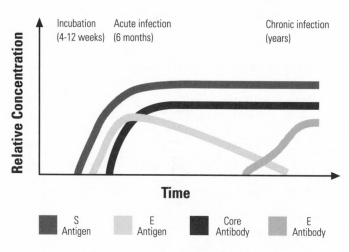

Reproduced with permission of GlaxoSmithKline

you can knock them off." Silent carriers have an increased chance of developing liver cancer from the age of 30–50, and must be monitored carefully with alpha-fetoprotein tests on a regular basis (usually every 6–12 months), especially for those like me who are older and/or those who have had the virus for many years.

Stages of liver disease

Liver fibrosis, with or without Chronic Active Infection—This stage is about apprehension for what the future may bring, as progressive liver injury is taking place, leading to liver scarring, otherwise known as fibrosis. Injury to liver cells is taking place on a microscopic level, causing inflammation.

What actually happens to the cells in this stage? The damage to hepatocytes starts affecting the protective **collagen** that circulates around and in between liver cells. Fibrosis is thought to occur when this collagen is altered or hindered from doing its job, leading to the development of tissue that is thicker and tougher than normal liver tissue. When this process continues unchecked, fibrotic tissue continues to develop, slowly spreading to smaller blood channels in the liver, where it causes hypertension, an arterial disease in which chronic high blood pressure is the primary symptom. As this process continues, new cells try to grow out from damaged areas but meet resistance from the tough, fibrotic tissue. As the new tissue grows within these limits, the liver slowly takes on the appearance of a cloth bag filled with tiny pellets. Sometimes doctors can feel the firm, bumpy surface of a cirrhotic liver on close examination of your upper right quadrant right under your right rib cage.

On your liver biopsy report you will notice that the pathologist grades liver fibrosis by either the Histological Activity Index (HAI) or **Knodell's Index** (see Appendix). This is a formulaic indicator of liver necrosis, fibrosis, and cirrhosis, and it is useful for choosing treatment or judging the effect of treatment.

Those of us with fibrosis experience a marked increase in fatigue, with gradual yet progressive interference of our normal diet and routines. Our liver's ability to deal with salt, sugar, fat, and protein is challenged. Ironically, sometimes people go into remission (no active replication and no detectable HBV DNA) when they are older or have suffered more severe liver damage. Blumberg held that HBV likes to keep us healthy throughout our most sexually active decades when we're most likely to be effective transmitters of the disease, and then it loses interest when our bodies slow down and our livers are damaged.

Cirrhosis, with or without Chronic Active Infection—In simple words this stage is similar to fibrosis, but here fibrosis has led to deeper, more extensive scarring along with irregular regeneration of the liver.

The word cirrhosis comes from Greek, and means tawny or orange, and was first described by a man named Laennec in 1826 as a condition in which the liver is "reduced to a third of its size with its external surface composed of a multitude of fawn-colored small grains varying in size from that of a millet seed to that of a hemp seed and on touch the liver gave the sensation of soft leather."

Cirrhosis is best understood as a progressive disease that is the result of a smoldering HBV infection with continuous intervals of scarring and regeneration. As mentioned above, it has three distinct characteristics: liver damage (necrosis), regeneration in an irregular fashion, and overall increase in fibrotic tissue, which causes malformation of liver lobules and surrounding blood vessels. HCV, alcohol abuse, congenital disorders, certain drugs, iron overload, obstructions of the bile duct, and autoimmune liver disease can also lead to cirrhosis.

Only 60 percent of those with cirrhosis actually experience symptoms, while the remaining 40 percent may never have the slightest idea that something is amiss. Your doctor may suspect cirrhosis if she takes many things into consideration, but final diagnosis can only be made after you've done your liver biopsy.

The development of cirrhosis may follow two or more decades of active HBV infection. Fortunately, with the help of antiviral treatment, this natural course of HBV has been altered in those who are diagnosed early and treated. It is also possible for those with chronic HBV to spontaneous clear HBsAg, yet the chance is quite small—only 1 percent per year. HBV infection continues to be a dynamic process, and long-term outcome is influenced by environmental factors like co-infection, treatment, immune response, host genetic factors, HBV mutations and genotypes, diet, and lifestyle.

Be vigilant about early signs of decompensation

In the presence of HBV the liver adapts—or compensates—by altering and adjusting its processes. Although the liver has an amazing capacity to multitask and regenerate, it does have its own threshold for what it can bear. When this threshold is exceeded we may experience a marked decline in liver functions, which usually signals the onset of cirrhosis. This is called decompensation. You may be decompensating if you:

○ Develop liver cell dysfunction (cancer or liver failure)
○ Have a buildup of ammonia or other toxins in your blood, leading to encephalopathy or sensory impairment
○ You become deeply jaundiced
○ Have evidence of vascular decompensation (**portal hypertension**)
○ Fluid accumulates in your abdomen (ascites) as witnessed by rapid weight gain (a pot belly, sometimes called *lordosis of cirrhosis*)
○ Bleed from your nose, gums, or skin
○ Suffer ruptured varices with massive gastrointestinal bleeding

If you are experiencing any or all of these symptoms you should see your doctor immediately or visit an emergency room. The other manifestations of cirrhosis which are commonly caused by liver cell failure are:

○ Decrease in overall health (poor appetite, fatigue, loss of muscle)
○ Rapid blood circulation, as witnessed by flushed face, red palms, swift heart rate, low blood pressure, bluish lips, or breathlessness)

○ Low grade fever
○ Bad breath, known as fetor hepaticus, a sickly sweet breath and a sign of impending complications and encephalopathy
○ Skin changes: spider veins, white spots on arms or buttocks
○ Changes in sex characteristics: loss of pubic hair, breast enlargement in men, diminished sex drive or impotency in men

Terminology for these stages keeps changing

Over the past few years the terminology used to describe these stages has changed. Why? Because our understanding of chronic liver disease has expanded, so much so that the terms previously used to describe them— chronic persistent hepatitis and chronic active hepatitis—have become too generic. Now we tend to say chronic hepatitis along with grade and stage of liver damage. For example, I am chronic active with stage three fibrosis. If you've already had your biopsy and don't know your status, ask your doctor to express it in these terms for you.

Your biopsy will determine the degree of inflammation. This measures the disease's activity. Then the stage of the disease will be determined by the amount of fibrosis that is present, ranging from none to bridging fibrosis and cirrhosis.

Your age has a lot to do with your chance of becoming chronic

The younger you are when you come into contact with HBV, the greater your likelihood of becoming chronic. Here is a quick statistical overview:

Chances of becoming chronic, by age

0–1 years	90%
1–5 years	40%
Teens/Adults	10%

As you can see, infants are at great risk for becoming chronic. For this reason it should be mandatory for pregnant women in the United States to be tested for HBV. In adolescents and adults, the virus usually keeps a low profile in order to pass unobserved, meaning that many of us remain entirely asymptomatic for years, even decades. It is important to remember that HBV is a slow-growing disease that causes damage over the course of decades.

Around 0.1–1 percent of cases of acute infection may result in **fulminant hepatitis** which, unfortunately, can be fatal without a **liver transplantation**. Those who are immunocompromised, meaning they have weak immune systems (transplant recipients and those with HIV), run a considerably higher risk of developing chronic infection.

IN A SENTENCE:

> *There are different stages of HBV depending on how long you've had the virus and how aggressively it is attacking your liver cells.*

living

Teaming with
Your Doctor

HBV REQUIRES that you and your doctor become a team. Due to widely varying strategies for treatment, potential side effects, uncertainties about treatment efficacy, and the prospect that HBV can become resistant to some drugs over time, doctors who treat HBV often ask for patient input.

Having to take responsibility for making decisions about your health may be a new idea for you, but it is actually part of an emerging doctor-patient paradigm. The old doctor-patient dynamic of Western medicine, in which M.D. stood for "medical deity," no longer exists. The Internet has very quickly become a major player for health care. Who could ever have imagined that we'd have come so far in just ten years? Health-related sites are the most commonly visited on the Internet (after pornography) and new technologies have enhanced the delicate doctor-patient relationship. Many HBV patients (and their families and partners) are gathering information to present to their doctors, a trend which is very likely to increase. Doctors are gradually being forced to take on the role of interpreters or analysts and slowly shed their identity as incontrovertible figureheads. Equipped with our own research, however, we are also prone to becoming disillusioned or challenging our medical professionals much more readily than in the past.

It's clear that we have the luxury of being able to concentrate on one disease, while doctors are responsible for knowing about dozens of diseases. It is virtually impossible for nonspecialists to keep up with innovation in every area of study. Disadvantaged by the limited amount of time to focus on our HBV, doctors are more likely to commit minor oversights that patients will catch and remember, thus it is not only likely but inevitable that patients will be switching doctors with greater frequency.

I left one doctor because he wouldn't agree to write an order for me to have an AFP (alpha feta protein) test, even though I'd been diagnosed with HBV for more than two years at that time. Through the nurse he sent back a message to me in the waiting room saying I didn't need it because the AFP was a cancer marker. I calmly told the nurse to tell him that HBV was the greatest cause of liver cancer worldwide, then turned and left. I never went back. You have to navigate a difficult and fine line between aggravation over a doctor's seemingly inconsequential oversights and exasperation over important lapses that can actually affect your health.

The dynamic that is developing takes a few more twists and turns but is potentially more effective and efficient. It seems to have the following configuration: doctor-patient-research-support group. Many HBV patients who accumulate information inevitably get lost in a thicket of research reports or studies, and eventually turn to online chat rooms, listservs, or support groups for more informed guidance and firsthand experience. The doctor, thus forced into a position as referee, is asked to judge the available information and his or her decision is much more public than it ever has been. One misstep can be publicized around the world to support groups in minutes.

If your doctor is inclined to scrunch up his face when you tell him about information from an online support group, you may want to take a few minutes to discuss his reaction openly with him. If you still feel his resistance, ask your doctor to provide a list of websites that have his stamp of approval. In fact, ask the doctor what his research resources are, and how you might access the same information. Essentially, it's a good idea to find a doctor that is open, curious, and passionate and, most importantly, one who isn't afraid to learn.

I like Sheree Martin's comment on doctors: "If you get the distinct impression that your doctor is annoyed with you, makes you feel like you're a bother, doesn't know how to treat your illnesses properly and covers that up by making *you* feel stupid, refuses to listen to new information that you try to share, won't let you get second opinions without feeling threatened, then you *need a new doctor*. After all, always remember, your doctor works *for you* and *with you*."

Teamwork: Helping your doctor help you

Once you find the perfect doctor for you, you may want to find ways to squeeze the most information out of him. Some of these tips may seem terribly obvious. Doctors, however, really do want you to hear them often so their information will rub off on you and become part of your routine. Recent statistics reveal that the average doctor's visit in the United States now lasts roughly 18 minutes (up from previous years). Clearly, you will need to prepare questions and organize your own information in advance in order to get the most out of your time allotment. Here are a few basic suggestions that will help you prepare for your visit:

- O Read about your condition and treatment options on reputable websites, in books and journals (see Resources), and familiarize yourself with medical terminology.
- O Get copies of charts and radiologists' reports.
- O Greet the doctor with a smile and ask how she is—doctors appreciate patients who show concern for their physicians' well-being.
- O Make sure to state the purpose (desired outcome) at the beginning of the visit, e.g., "I'm hoping to choose a HBV treatment strategy today," or, "I want to better understand my options now that I've done my biopsy," or, "I'd like to brainstorm with you about how to minimize my fatigue." Many doctors are trained to ask as a standard practice what a patient wants to accomplish in the visit and plan the visit accordingly.
- O Be honest and tell the doctor how you really feel—don't censor your responses. However, since time is limited, try to give concrete, objective information with clear time frames. One way to do this is by keeping good lists of the following information:
    - ⇨ Your symptoms and their duration
    - ⇨ Your former doctors and their contact information
    - ⇨ Your allergies, including those to medicines. Be specific.
    - ⇨ Your medical history and hospitalizations
    - ⇨ Your family medical history
- O Buy a notebook for keeping these lists, and review them in the waiting room so that you don't have to search for them while you're with the doctor, wasting valuable time.
- O Ask the doctor to repeat and further elaborate on topics you don't fully understand.

O Don't be embarrassed to discuss personal details like your stools or sexual issues.

O Decide which of your concerns is most important, and bring it up with the doctor first.

O Ask the doctor if there is a nurse who can further explain things to you if you feel he or she is rushed or unable to answer in a way that is easy for you to understand.

O Ask for any brochures, pamphlets, or videos that they might have on hand—some pharmaceutical companies publish excellent information for patients.

O If at all possible, don't cancel your appointments at the last moment—this will discourage the doctor from spending extra time with you the next time you have an appointment.

O Take a friend if your memory is uneven, if you are experiencing brain fog, or if your child is the patient, but don't let your friend talk on your behalf. You can also take a small tape recorder with you.

O Ask the best way to funnel postvisit questions back to the doctor. In particular, ask if the office makes use of e-mail, or if there is a nurse triage hotline available.

O If you do not speak or understand your doctor's language fully and fluently, bring a close friend (not a relative) who can help translate.

What not to do

The bulleted information above is a basic list of things that we should do to help our physicians. On the other hand, there are also quite a few things that patients do to irritate their health care professionals. After conducting an informal survey of friends and colleagues in the medical field, Patrice Al-Saden, RN, and I have recognized a pattern of responses that highlight frictions between doctors and certain patients. Do you recognize yourself in any of these items? If so, try apologizing on your next visit. You really can't afford to be on a doctor's bad side.

Top Ten Things People Do To Bother Healthcare Workers

1. Failure to show up for appointments or cancel appointments in advance

2. Interrupting the nurse or doctor with a call just to inform him or her that you are not feeling well and don't feel like coming to your scheduled appointment

3. Complaining to the nurse or doctor about the high cost of health care

4. Asking for advice and then choosing to disregard it
5. Knowingly jeopardizing your health.
6. Thinking there is a pill to cure everything and refusing to leave the office without a prescription
7. Expressing frustration when the doctor or nurse is late and expecting that the doctor or nurse spend an unlimited amount of time with them, thus making the doctor or nurse late for the next patient
8. Thinking that medical professionals are perfect and superhuman—forgetting that medical professionals have significant others, children, and lives, as well as the happiness and problems that come along with all of that
9. Demanding that health care professionals never make mistakes or errors in judgment
10. Wanting answers to questions that are sometimes unanswerable

IN A SENTENCE:

Do your homework before your visit to your hepatologist and remember that you have equal responsibility in determining the best treatment for you.

learning

What Does
My Liver Do?

A JACK-OF-ALL-TRADES, the liver carries out over
500 functions for your body. However, the liver's main jobs are
to convert food to energy, store this energy in the form of glucose or glycogen, and filter waste and toxic substances from
your blood.

The liver is the body's largest organ, making up roughly 1\50th
of your body weight. It is divided into areas called lobes, and is
shaped somewhat like a triangle. It rests mostly under your right
rib cage, though a small part of the bottom of your liver extends
past your rib cage. This overall area is often referred to by medical professionals as your upper right quadrant.

Oxygen-enriched blood is carried to the liver by the portal
vein, which pumps in blood from the stomach and intestines,
and the hepatic artery, which brings in blood from the heart and
lungs. Two major conduits take fluids away from your liver: the
hepatic veins drain blood, while the bile ducts transport bile to
your gallbladder. Amazingly, a healthy liver is able to filter about
a liter of blood per minute, making it a star performer of our
immune systems.

When your doctor taps on the area of your abdomen above
your liver, she may hear a deep or full sound. Sometimes your
doctor can tell if you have liver damage just by the sound that

reverberates from her gentle tapping. Your liver does not feel pain (although the protective capsule around it does), so your liver may not let you know it is sick until 75 percent of its function has been lost.

Here is a more specific list of the liver's functions.

Regulates energy metabolism. Your liver maintains sufficient levels of **carbohydrates** and fats to provide constant energy to other tissues, for example, it utilizes glucose for energy and is a storehouse for glycogen, which it breaks down on demand when our bodies need energy. Many people don't know that the liver also makes use of fats for energy and stores others for later use. The liver also regulates your **cholesterol** and triglyceride levels. Given that the liver is a veritable power generator, we can understand how the slowing of our carbohydrate metabolism and lack of adequate glycogen storage means that fatigue is the most noticeable symptom when our livers are impaired or inflamed.

Manufactures new body proteins and breaks them down. This helps maintain constant levels in our tissue and blood. When the liver has a hard time juggling all these proteins, we can develop swelling, muscle wasting, or clotting problems. Sometimes a lack of proper proteins can cause us to bruise, cut, or scrape more easily, and it can take us longer to heal. Others may experience gingivitis (bleeding gums).

Makes bile, which helps us digest fats and is essential for digestion. It is also a vehicle for excreting numerous toxins from chemicals and drugs. When we don't process bile efficiently, we can experience malabsorption, diarrhea, and jaundice.

Acts as a filter to clear the blood of both toxic and nontoxic substances. For example, your liver converts ammonia to nontoxic **urea** so it can be passed from your system via your kidneys, and it transforms hormones, drugs, and other chemicals into by-products for excretion. The liver also tries its best to metabolize alcohol. When the liver can't keep up, alcohol and toxins can stay in your body for more extended periods, further damaging cells. If not enough ammonia is removed from our blood we can develop brain fog or encephalopathy from brain swelling.

Regenerates its own tissue when damaged or when a section is surgically removed. The liver is the only organ in our body which can actually grow back if damaged or if an entire section is removed. This amazing and intense reparative metabolic activity begins within 6 hours of partial surgical removal of the liver, gradually resulting in restoration of both the original liver mass and its lobular structure. It is even more amazing that the liver's regenerative capacity is unaffected by repeated resection or damage. The exact mechanism of this regeneration is still unknown, but several enzymes and hormones released in the blood play an important role.

Governs the activity of drugs in the body. When the liver can't keep track of the drugs in your body, these drugs can build up and have an even more potent effect on the rest of your body. For this reason it is important to discuss any medications (both prescription and over-the-counter) with your doctor, and remind her every visit about the drugs you are taking. Be careful when you are taking HIV antivirals and antifungals with names that end in "-azole." Common steroids, some antibiotics, and anticonvulsants should also be monitored very carefully. You must check each drug for its interaction on the liver and adjust its dose if required. One should be careful with herbal supplements as well. Obviously, recreational drugs are out of the question for those with liver disease.

Regulates hormones, especially steroids and sex hormones. Hormonal irregularity may only develop with the onset of cirrhosis, but can cause breast enlargement and impotence in men or genital atrophy in women and loss of libido in both sexes.

Regulates blood clotting by manufacturing most of our clotting factors. Liver cells are the manufacturing center of elements that regulate blood clotting. As a consequence, a damaged liver results in prolongation of clotting time. A vitamin K deficiency can also prolong clotting, as it is also stored in the liver.

IN A SENTENCE:

> The liver has an extraordinary array of important tasks to carry out such as filtering toxins and regulating energy and hormones.

DAY 7

living

Managing Your Fatigue

GETTING A handle on HBV symptoms is a bit like trying to wrestle a herd of cats—they're all over the place. Some of us don't experience any symptoms at all, while others seem to experience all of them. Some symptoms seem to come and go at intervals while other show up every day like clockwork. Unfortunately, it can be difficult to find a doctor that will deal with your fatigue. If you sense that your doctor isn't interested in addressing it directly, ask her for a referral to a nutritionist, therapist, or physical therapist. Or, try a new doctor.

You may not have any symptoms at all

If you're wondering what I'm talking about right now, you may be asymptomatic. Forty percent of us are. That means that although you have HBV in your body, you are experiencing none of the symptoms that pester the rest of us. Some of us can be asymptomatic for years at a time and then experience a flare, which is an increase in liver enzymes and perhaps even HBV DNA, causing more acute symptoms that can last for weeks or months.

Fatigue has many guises

Fatigue is undoubtedly the most common symptom of hepatitis B, and it presents itself differently in every person. It can be mild and indistinguishable from tiredness, like the way you feel when you're stuck in a meeting with a boring speaker, or it can be so incapacitating that you feel like you can't get out of bed. It can be localized, seeming to emanate from your lower abdomen, like a bout of stomach flu, or it can take over your whole body and limbs. If your ALT levels are high you may even feel like you're suffering from a bout of botulism, or like you have a hangover. Bad fatigue reminds me of how I felt in the recovery room at the hospital after anesthesia—poisoned and debilitated.

Susan Grant's experience is typical of what severe fatigue does to our outlook on life: "I remember my husband and I were shopping and I told him to just buy a small tube of toothpaste because I truly believed that I would not live long enough to use a big tube! That was 12 years ago. I did get better, but the fatigue is worse than anything."

About half of us seem to experience the most fatigue in the morning, while the other half experience fatigue at the end of the day. Some of us look like we've been partying all night even though we've had 9 hours of sleep. Others wear their fatigue beneath happy and healthy façades. Personally I dread 3:30 to 5:30 P.M. I have to splash cold water on my face and do breathing exercises to make it to the end of the working day. Of course it should be remembered that even perfectly healthy people experience fatigue, and not all of our fatigue is due to HBV.

Fatigue brings about brain fog

Fatigue isn't just physical; it's mental too. Sometimes intellectual fatigue can seem more challenging and annoying than physical fatigue, as it can be coupled with what people with hepatitis call brain fog. Technically, brain fog is due to mild swelling of the brain or a buildup of toxins. In medical terms it is referred to as encephalopathy when it becomes much more pronounced.

What a relief it was for me to hear that term the first time! It instantly validated the emotional turmoil I'd been experiencing for years but hadn't connected to HBV. I thought I must have been slightly dyslexic or have attention deficit disorder. Studies show that when the immune system is fighting a virus, it releases substances called cytokines and neuropeptides that interrupt blood flow in the brain. This is a normal process for fighting viral infection.

However, when the body is fighting off a chronic viral infection, it releases these substances all the time at the most inopportune moments.

With brain fog thoughts become fuzzy. Ideas resist translation into words. It feels as if you have awakened to a phone call in the middle of the night and you struggle to get the words out, although some of us feel that way for hours at a time. It can be embarrassing and depressing, even frightening for those of us with jobs that require nimble thinking or operations involving memory. I keep small Post-it notes on my desk at work. Every time I have a task I write it on one of the notes and I line the notes up on the edge of my desk. It works. Thankfully, some of us manage to get a good laugh out of it. We share stories about how brain fog can think you make like this.

Fatigue isn't always due to HBV

Although HBV is probably the most likely cause of our fatigue, we shouldn't assume that it is the only culprit. Anemia, mononucleosis, allergies, or hypothyroidism, among others, could be contributing factors, as well as stress. A poor diet, cigarettes, drugs, or alcohol can really take their toll. The following are just a few of the possible tests that a doctor may run to rule out other contributing factors: complete blood count (CBC) to check for anemia, chemistry panel to check kidney function and electrolyte imbalance, thyroid tests such as TRH (hypothalamus) or TSH (pituary), testosterone level for men or DHEA for women. Your doctor may even decide to rule out mononucleosis or sexually transmitted diseases (STDs). Some test blood sugar levels or adrenal insufficiency. Medications can be to blame for excess fatigue, as well as sleep apnea or snoring. Don't be too quick to dismiss any possible causes.

In my case, after drinking unpurified lake water over a two-week vacation in Canada, I insisted that my primary physician check into parasites as a possible explanation for my unusual fatigue, irregular bowel movements, headaches, and tightness in my chest. An online article about how people with liver disease were more susceptible to parasites had tipped me off. My doctor at that time laughed at my homegrown diagnosis but wrote out the order anyway and we made a symbolic bet about the outcome. He wasn't laughing when the test came back positive for what was a rather unpleasant and unwelcome hitchhiker in my body. But, the lesson learned was crucial: don't be so focused on your virus that you can't see the forest for the trees; HBV isn't always going to be the only cause of your fatigue.

You look good and feel terrible

One of the greatest challenges about having HBV is that sometimes you don't look sick. In fact, you can look downright healthy. For this reason, friends can get offended if you put off too many invitations to go out to dinner or drinks. Inevitably it is hard to explain to those without HBV why you look great and feel terrible, and you're not always going to be convincing. You will hear comments like, "You should get more sleep," "Don't work so hard," or a personal favorite, "Are you taking better care of yourself now?" Looking great and feeling terrible is one of the hallmarks of hepatitis.

On the other hand, sometimes you will feel great and look terrible. Once in a while, when I'm merrily brewing my first cup of watered down decaf in the office, someone will look at me and say "Hey, did you have a late night last night?" This is especially hard to hear when you've just had nine hours of sleep and feel pumped up.

What can I do to minimize fatigue?

Fortunately, we can learn to minimize, or at least manage, the fatigue we experience during the day. Our success will depend on our enzyme levels and other markers, but we can try some of the following strategies that have proved useful for others who I've interviewed.

Sleep

Getting a good night's sleep is essential for those with HBV. It is generally recommended to get at least eight hours of sleep every night. I know this sounds self-evident, even for healthy people. But how many of us actually manage to get eight hours every night? We don't seem to have time to sleep.

Keep regular hours. In addition to getting at least your full eight hours, those with HBV can maximize sleep's restorative effect by going to bed at the same time every night. Though we don't quite know why, this seems to have a significant effect on mitigating fatigue. If you find this hard to believe, try to keep a regular schedule for a month, then go back to your old ways. You'll be surprised at how much better you felt when you kept regular hours.

Of course this may put a cramp in your social life, as if the no-alcohol edict wasn't enough. A ten o'clock bedtime may also make you feel like you're ten years old again. My closest friends know I turn into Cinderella quite early, and I start yawning in a very annoying way at about 9:30 P.M.

So I schedule activities in order to be in bed by at least 10:30 P.M. and I find that if I get to bed any later I wake tired and stay tired all day. My hours are so regular now that even a half-hour delay has an effect on me.

Block out light. I can't seem to sleep in a room with any light at all. I was so frustrated that I put up lined curtains like the ones you find in hotels. Some people prefer to use sleep masks.

Use white noise. I have other friends who insist on having white noise to aid their sleep. It's especially effective if you live on a noisy street or have a barking dog nearby.

Dine early and/or eat lighter meals more frequently. Try making your lunchtime meal your largest meal of the day, and eat smaller meals more frequently. If you have difficulty sleeping or feel that you're sleeping too lightly, check to make sure you're not eating too late in the evening.

Cut out caffeine. This works like a charm. You may think this is cruel, especially since you've already had to give up those other stimulants and depressants. There are so few drinks without caffeine that this really limits you. Substitute decaf or herbal tea whenever possible. If you just cannot do without at least some caffeine, try and limit your caffeine intake to the morning hours.

Buy a good mattress. Getting a good mattress is a critical part of getting better sleep.

Get exercise. You are going to get tired of hearing this suggestion.

Eat a snack with tryptophan, magnesium, and thiamin. A mug of warm skim milk, or a handful of almonds, or slice of turkey can raise levels of serotonin in your brain and may help to induce sleep.

Eat well and take vitamins

We will discuss diet more in depth in Week 2, but remember that your diet is critical for minimizing fatigue and giving your liver a break. Cut down on saturated fats, red meat, excess sugar, and salt. Try to eat more dark green vegetables. Vitamins may help too, but don't go overboard. Try a children's vitamin without iron. Avoid megavitamins, as some are fat-soluble and can be stored in the liver and become toxic.

Vitamin B_{12}. During a particularly tough bout of fatigue, a shot of vitamin B_{12} may provide temporary relief. One study found that a B_{12} tablet dissolved under the tongue had the same effect. A B vitamin complex is a good idea.

Other strategies can help beat fatigue

Drink filtered water. Have a good filtration system installed in your home, and drink at least 8 glasses of water per day. Try not to wait until the evening to drink all that fluid, as you will interrupt your deep sleep with trips to the bathroom. If you insist on drinking caffeine, chase it with the same amount of purified water. Drinking water is especially important if you are on Interferon, as it could help alleviate some of the side effects. Some find it helpful to drink a mixture of 1 part lemonade to 3 parts water to make all that liquid more appetizing. See Month 11 for more ideas about how to keep hydrated.

Listen to music. Some Mozart and a hot water bottle over your liver is a winning combination.

Take a nap. A 20-minute power nap can do wonders for you during the day. If you don't have an office with a door, you may be able to find a quiet place at work, as some companies set aside rooms for women who are lactating and need to express milk. Let your boss know that you're using your lunch hour and not company time.

Address the stress in your life. Many people with HBV say that stress is one of the leading causes of fatigue. Addressing it quickly is wise.

Have a sauna or a hot bath. One of the quickest ways to head off fatigue is to get your circulation going by heating your body up a bit. A sauna or a hot bath makes your fatigue melt away.

You've probably realized by now that fatigue isn't caused by one single thing in your body, and it isn't treated by a single medication or change in habits. You will want to weave as many of these suggestions as you can into your daily regimen.

IN A SENTENCE:

> *Fatigue is the most common HBV symptom, however altering your diet and adapting your routine can minimize its effect.*

learning

Slaying the Dragon:
Your First Liver Biopsy

WHEN MY doctor first told me I would need to have a biopsy, I wasn't too concerned. I imagined that it would be performed with full anesthesia and that there would be an incision. I imagined that a piece of my liver, the size of a dime, would be removed, and that I'd wake up relaxed and refreshed. Later I was horrified to hear that it would be performed while I was awake. Awake? I'm the guy who gets lightheaded just thinking about giving blood. I rationalized my way out of the biopsy by convincing myself it wouldn't make a difference in my treatment, therefore it was useless.

Reality check: the procedure *is* essential for keeping track of your liver's health, the tiny sliver of liver removed is incredibly thin and just a few inches long, and the actual procedure takes only a minute or so from start to finish. Despite this knowledge, I still waited three years before I worked up the courage. I'm not proud of that fact. And what is worse, by delaying the biopsy, I delayed a critical period of my treatment.

You will probably be asked to undergo a biopsy before treatment

A biopsy can help to make a more specific diagnosis by determining the severity of the disease and the extent of scarring that may have occurred. It can also act as a screening process for liver cancer or other liver diseases that can develop from medications.

In general, however, patients with normal liver enzymes are not usually asked to undergo a liver biopsy, except in certain circumstances. A biopsy is the only way to detect at the cellular level what damage has already occurred and is still occurring in your liver. Although it may seem hard to believe, liver enzyme tests don't necessarily match what's going on inside of the liver. Sometimes those of us with severe cirrhosis have normal enzymes. For example, I have normal enzymes even though I suffer advanced fibrosis. Given that I follow a strict diet, exercise every day, and don't smoke, drink, or stress out too much, I was convinced beforehand that my liver was fine. I was wrong. A biopsy will let the doctor know once and for all how damaged your liver is, if at all.

Biopsies aren't usually as painful as you might think

For obvious and understandable reasons, many of you are also thinking about delaying or even avoiding this procedure. You hear or read horror stories of excruciatingly painful biopsies, needles as big as harpoons stuck into one's side. I had visions of some weapon out of a *Terminator* movie.

The truth is that, after the fact, most of us say it wasn't nearly as bad as we thought it would be—me included. Anticipation of the procedure is definitely worse than the procedure itself. You are taking the first and possibly most important step in taking care of your liver. The actual biopsy takes only a minute. You will receive local anesthesia beforehand, and if you request one, you may be given a mild sedative to take the edge off.

You will need to give blood a week before your biopsy

Here is how the procedure usually takes place for a percutaneous biopsy, which is the most common method. You will be asked to go in for the following blood tests about a week before the procedure:

Prothrombin time-international normalized ratio and partial thrombo-plastin time (PTT and PT)

This test measures the time it takes for blood to clot. Blood clotting requires vitamin K and a protein made by the liver. Liver cell damage and bile flow obstruction can both interfere with proper blood clotting.

Platelet count

Platelets are small blood cells and are involved in the clotting process. In chronic liver diseases, the **platelet count** usually falls only after cirrhosis has developed, and can be abnormal in many other conditions other than liver diseases.

Hemoglobin

Measures the total amount of hemoglobin, which is the iron-containing pigment in red blood cells.

Your doctor will tell you to avoid aspirin and NSAIDs (nonsteroidal anti-inflammatory drugs like ibuprofen—see Month 9 for a complete listing)—for one week before the biopsy, and **anticoagulants** should also be stopped. Let your doctor know if you take insulin. It may be necessary to stop or adjust medications before your test.

You will be asked to fast from around midnight the night before the procedure. The doctor or nurse will explain the procedure to you. You will sign a consent form stating that you have been told about the procedure and its possible complications. An intravenous line (IV) will most likely be started; perhaps some more blood will be drawn.

The day of the biopsy

The doctor may feel your liver, tap over it, and ask you to breathe in and hold it. Your doctor is trying to find the borders of your liver. They are making a mental outline of it. Doing this helps them pick the best spot to stick the liver. Sometimes they use a portable ultrasound machine that will outline the liver for them and they may mark your skin with a marker. When the spot is chosen, a local anesthetic is injected to the skin. Smile and encourage your doctor to use plenty. This will sting or burn for about 15 seconds. A nick in the skin is made with a scalpel and a needle, (yes it's long) and is inserted usually between the 8th and 9th rib. You may feel pressure at this point. Some doctors use a kind of automatic gun.

The liver feels no pain. However, the membrane surrounding the liver, called Glisson's capsule, does have nerve endings and does feel pain. When the needle passes through this membrane you may feel a momentary twinge of discomfort, or feel queasy about the idea of a needle entering the liver. The actual biopsy stick lasts a fraction of a second. My hepatologist put the sample in a jar and let me see it. It was paper-thin and a few inches long. I appreciated this insight.

You can request a sedative before the procedure

You can request a mild sedative like Versed, Valium, or Midozolam beforehand, and it may be given either through your IV or in your buttock. I took the shot and, ironically, that shot involved more pain than the ensuing biopsy. In any case, think about whether you might want it in advance, and let the doctor know long before he or she is ready to perform the biopsy. Some people prefer to undergo the procedure without sedating medicine.

Your right shoulder may ache during the procedure and for up to 48 hours afterwards. This is called referred pain. The right shoulder shares a nerve tract with the area of the liver biopsy, so it is possible to feel a dull ache around or above your shoulder blade.

You may be asked to exhale and hold your breath when the doctor takes the actual liver sample. You will be asked to hold very still.

You won't be able to move for a few hours after the biopsy

For 1–4 hours after the biopsy you will be asked to lie on your right side. Since the biopsy leaves a tiny puncture wound in the liver, there is a high risk of bleeding. Lying on your right side with a pressure dressing (a big bandage) puts the weight of your liver against your rib cage, creating a natural seal. This helps promote clotting and prevent bleeding.

The nurse will check your vital signs often (blood pressure, pulse, temperature, respiration) and ask you how you are feeling every so often. You may be offered some pain medication if you feel you need it. You will be allowed to eat, drink, and sit up after the 1–4 hours. In general, hospitals will discharge after a few hours, while a few choose to schedule biopsies in the late afternoon so you can stay overnight in the hospital for monitoring. Eventually, you will be able to go home with your designated driver. Don't plan on going back to work or shopping or attending a wedding. Just let yourself off the hook and take it easy for a day. You've earned it.

You should not remove your pressure dressing until the following morning, at which time you can take a shower or bath. Then you can pat yourself on the back. You've passed the HBV initiation.

There are other, less common methods for performing liver biopsies

Sometimes doctors will choose to use an ultrasound or CT to help determine the best entry point for the needle. Some doctors use this method by default, while others use it for children or patients who are either overweight or who have undersized or hidden livers.

Still other methods are utilized for those with advanced liver disease or bleeding problems. **Laparoscopy** uses a thin, lighted tube that passes through a small incision in the abdomen. With this technique, small pieces of liver may be taken from more than one area of the liver.

Transjugular biopsies entail passing a special catheter through an internal jugular vein in the neck. Sometime this procedure is performed by a radiologist when the patient has advanced scarring, a problem with blood clotting (**coagulopathy**) or ascites.

Lastly, surgical biopsies are carried out while the patient is undergoing abdominal surgery. If you have another surgery on the horizon, this may seem like a great way to avoid unnecessary stress, as you can have the procedure done while you're already having surgery for a different reason.

Complications are quite rare

Only about one in 5,000 people experiences some kind of complication from liver biopsy. Bleeding from the site of the puncture can occur, but does so in less than 1 percent of patients. Other complications could involve a punctured lung, kidney, gallbladder, intestine, or artery in the liver. A punctured gallbladder could, for example, lead to a leak of bile fluids that could cause **peritonitis**. Very rarely does a patient have a complication requiring hospitalization. All the same, it is a good idea not to stray far from home or hospital for at least two weeks after the procedure.

Try to stay within reasonable distance of a hospital in the unlikely event that complications arise. Some people I interviewed even wisely recommend carrying a note with you informing others that you've recently had a biopsy.

Your biopsy is then graded

There are a few different grading systems for grading what is known as the Histology Activity Index (HAI) of your biopsy. The original index, known as the Knodell Score (1981), was modified by Ludwig (1993) and Ishak (1995). In the United States most are given two grades: measurement of inflammation or necrosis, which is assigned a grade, and scarring or fibrosis, which is given a stage. Broadly speaking, there are four stages of scarring and fibrosis, and the individual scores are added to determine a HAI score. See resources for an abridged explanation of these grades and stages.

Your biopsy is graded much like ice skaters at the World Championships. One judge says it's a perfect six and another will insist it's a 5.5. In other words, it's a subjective system. Pathologists may evaluate the same slide differently on subsequent readings, or different pathologists may grade the same sample with different scores. More importantly, these scores are sometimes misunderstood or misinterpreted.

For that reason, if things are unclear or if there are doubts, it is wise to get a second opinion of your reading. Ask to have your slides—your liver sample sandwiched between sheets of glass—sent to another lab or doctor for the reading. But, do make sure the slides are returned.

The results of your biopsy may surprise you

I hope that you will be pleasantly surprised to discover that you have minimal or no scarring or inflammation. Setting your expectations quite low is healthy when you're waiting for biopsy results, since your actual level of energy and overall health is not an indication of what your biopsy will look like. Make sure that you get a copy of the biopsy results, and make another appointment to discuss the implications of these results with your hepatologist.

My former GI specialist called me up at work a few days after my first biopsy and said simply, "It doesn't look very good, but it could be worse. See you in six months," and hung up before I could catch my breath. There was no effort on his part to explain the grading and staging and no discussion of next steps or possible treatment strategies. Although I respected his brain, he never got another call from me.

You can feel proud about completing your first biopsy

The prospect of having a liver biopsy is much more frightening than the reality. But since you've now met this challenge head-on, you should feel proud about your accomplishment. Treat yourself to a day in a spa or a weekend in the country. Congratulations on completing this essential step in treating HBV.

IN A SENTENCE:

Having a biopsy is not as painful as it sounds, and it is absolutely essential for determining the exact condition of your liver.

FIRST-WEEK MILESTONE

By the end of your first week you've taken the first crucial steps toward regaining your health as quickly as possible, as you have now:

○ VERIFIED YOUR DIAGNOSIS WITH TESTS AND A BIOPSY.

○ LEARNED ABOUT FINDING A GOOD SPECIALIST.

○ EDUCATED YOURSELF ABOUT THE BASICS OF HBV.

○ FOUND WAYS TO CONNECT TO THE WORLDWIDE HBV SUPPORT NETWORK.

○ READ ABOUT SOME OF HBV'S MOST COMMON SYMPTOMS.

Nutrition Basics

WHEN YOU have HBV, it sometimes seems like you're not allowed to eat anything. When I was younger, I used to call it the no-fun diet. The world we live in likes exaggerated flavors and saturated fats, and new packaged foods in the supermarket seem to be made for some superhuman race yet to be born. One has to look long and far to find a prepared food or bottled drink that doesn't have sugar, caffeine, food coloring, alcohol, or artificial sweeteners. You practically need a chemistry degree to read and understand the label on a package of hot dogs. Everyone has a pet conspiracy theory, and mine is that alien infiltrators are posing as food engineers and taking over our big corporate food laboratories, concocting tasty and easy to prepare meals that hide harmful chemicals, hormones, radiation, DNA engineering, and saturated fats. All this with the devious goal of weakening our immune system, shortening our life expectancy, and taking over our fair nation. Yes, I know this sounds a bit silly, but unfortunately in this age of frankenfoods and irradiation, it doesn't sound like science fiction anymore.

Consequently, when you feel like the only aisle you can shop in is the fresh produce aisle (and even then you're not completely at ease!), going to the supermarket can be a demoralizing or depressing experience. The first thing we need to do after learning nutrition basics is to concentrate on phasing out unhealthy things (see Month 2). Then we need to slowly phase in wholesome and nourishing foods (see Month 11). But first, knowing a little bit about nutrition will help us get to a healthier place. The more you know, the more you're likely to eat right and give your liver a break.

It's good to understand the basic building blocks of nutrition

We all know that there are basic food groups: protein, carbohydrates, and fat. But do we all know what they do once they are in our bodies? I was lucky enough to grow up in a home with a nutritionist who always coupled food names with their nutritional content. My mother would always call after us, "Eat your banana—you need potassium" or "How are you going to get your vitamin A if you don't eat your carrots?" Although we didn't seem to pay much attention at the time, her insistence is paying off now. Unfortunately, very few of us have learned the basics at home or at school—not even our doctors.

Your liver is a nutrient factory and warehouse

As mentioned before, your liver is your command control center: it metabolizes, converts, stores, and distributes nutrients to our other organs, and does its best to make sure that we have a constant energy supply. For example, the liver converts glycogen into glucose for energy and cholesterol into bile so it can be eliminated from our system. And the liver has a real talent for handling proteins.

Proteins are broken down into amino acids by our livers

Proteins are essential for our health. Our livers, with help from our intestines and pancreas, break down these proteins into dozens of amino acids that carry out a wide range of important bodily functions. They maintain tissue health and repair DNA when it is damaged, but they also produce components of antibodies to help the immune system. While our bodies create a perfect dozen of these amino acids, we must get 9 others, called essential amino acids, from the food we eat.

Most of us are aware of the primary sources of protein—meat, fish, dairy products, and eggs. Contrary to popular belief, we don't have to eat meat to get enough protein in our diet. If you're eating red meat, you're also getting a lot of fat. Yes, even lean meat: just one ounce still has 10 grams of fat. And that's before you slap on the steak sauce. Few people know that we can also get protein from plants such as soybeans, legumes, and even seaweed. Dark, leafy green vegetables like spinach, broccoli, and kale, for example, all have protein. In fact, all vegetables have protein to some degree.

For those with minimal or moderate liver damage, a good steady supply of protein throughout the day is ideal so we can help our livers maintain consistent energy levels. We may think that protein is so good that we need to consume a lot of it. The intestines produce small amounts of ammonia during the digestion process, and normally it is converted into urea and excreted by the kidneys. However, severe liver damage makes it hard for the liver to successfully synthesize proteins, so those with cirrhosis and liver failure may need to limit their intake and eat more vegetable and milk proteins rather than meat proteins (especially red meats). When our livers are damaged and we eat too much protein, ammonia can build up and affect our nervous system and cause brain fog. High levels of ammonia in those with cirrhosis can also, unfortunately, lead to coma. Studies show that too much protein may even cause some drugs to be converted into toxins. The same holds true for excessive amino acids, so avoid taking large doses of amino acid supplements.

Twenty to thirty percent of your daily intake should be in protein, and depending on your weight, this can translate to between 50–100 grams daily.

Carbohydrates provide us with energy

Carbohydrates, also known as starches or carbs, are converted to sugar in the body. Carbohydrates are fuel for your body, and should give you more than half the calories you need in your balanced diet. Breads, cereals, and grains are the main players here, but carbs can also be found in fruits, vegetables, and dairy products. Carbohydrates are actually present in all food except meat and meat alternatives.

The liver breaks down carbohydrates into glycogen and glucose when we need energy. Your blood then transports this energy to every cell in your body for energy. A limited quantity of glycogen is stored in your liver as an energy reserve until it's needed. Carbs can be simple or complex. Simple carbohydrates refer to a single sugar molecule or two sugars linked together. Complex carbohydrates are long chains of sugars linked together. You can find complex carbs in whole grain bread and pasta, beans, and brown rice, among other things.

People with hepatitis should make an effort to eat more complex carbs than simple ones, as hepatitis challenges the liver's ability to regulate blood sugar levels. Ironically, some people I interviewed were diagnosed with hepatitis B after going to the doctor expecting to be diagnosed with diabetes. Others with both HBV and diabetes say that their diabetic diet seems to help keep some of the HBV symptoms like fatigue and brain fog at bay.

The liver has a love/hate relationship with fats

We all know that excess fat in our diet can clog our arteries. But not too many of us know that the wrong kind of fats also weigh on the liver and can exacerbate our hepatitis symptoms. All fats are made up of carbon chains with hydrogen atoms attached to each carbon. The good fats have gaps between hydrogen atoms so that our bodies can use them for various biochemical functions like transporting vitamins throughout the body. These gaps act like joints so that the fat can be bent to adjust to our body's requirements. These are called unsaturated fats, and we sometimes hear them referred to as monounsaturated and polyunsaturated fats. Monounsaturated oils like canola, olive, and peanut oil have one gap, while polyunsaturated oils like flax, corn, sesame, and sunflower oil have two or more gaps.

Saturated, trans, and hydrogenated oils, however, have no gaps and are unbendable. For this reason they don't lend themselves to carrying out important cellular activities. What is more, they even impede our body's ability to process good oils, potentially leading to chronic disease and coronary heart disease. No more than 10 percent of our total daily caloric intake should be from saturated fat, and no more than 30 percent from any kind of fat. It is pretty safe to say that most Americans eat nearly twice this recommended amount. People with liver problems do not have this luxury, but that is definitely a good thing. By being forced to take care of our livers, we can also care for our hearts. See Month 2 for more about hydrogenated oils. Here is a quick summary of fats to eat and fats to avoid:

Good fats
> Fish oils, nut oils, seed oils, olive oil, butter (in moderation), evening primrose oil, and those containing the essential omega-6 and omega-3 oils

Foods containing good fats
> Seeds, avocados, cereals, legumes, olives, soybeans, fish, and most nuts

Bad fats
> Hydrogenated and partially hydrogenated fats, refined vegetable oils, and saturated fats, coconut oil, palm kernel oil

Foods containing bad fats

> Fried foods, processed foods, chips and snacks, animal skins, margarine and butter, mayonnaise, and salad dressings

Our bodies have a love/hate relationship with cholesterol

We've been taught that cholesterol is a bad thing, but, like fat, there's good cholesterol and bad cholesterol. We get cholesterol from some foods, but our liver also produces it on its own. This is a prime example of our liver's ingenuity, since it both manufactures cholesterol and removes it simultaneously via tiny receptors attached to our liver cells. When we eat too much fat we clog these receptors, causing our cholesterol levels to rise. High fat intake can make those who have both diabetes and HBV even more susceptible to other problems like eye, kidney, and nerve disease.

Low-density lipoproteins (LDL) are responsible for most of the cholesterol deposits in our arteries. We can lower our LDL levels if we monitor our intake of saturated fat and increase fiber in our diet. The normal range of LDL level is 60–180 mg/dl (milligrams per deciliter). **High-density lipoproteins (HDL)**, on the other hand, are good fats that actually remove cholesterol from our circulatory system. The normal range of HDL is, for males, 29–62 mg/dl, and for females, 34–82 mg/dl. You can use the following trick to memorize which is good and bad: LDL is lousy and HDL is happy.

Medium chain triglycerides (MCT) are tiny fat globules and are most often found in coconut oil and butter. MCT is absorbed and converted into energy more quickly because they are shorter than longer chain fatty acids. Although it may be true that MCT provides some health benefits like providing quick energy, building muscle, and stimulating insulin production, there are conflicting opinions. Consuming too much MCT is not recommended for people with hepatitis because it can give us cramps and, because of its saturated fat content, it can also promote heart disease.

Ask your doctor if it might be a good idea to gauge your fat intake and risk for heart disease by having a lipid panel and or cholesterol check done along with your next liver panel.

Vitamins and minerals

When you were smaller you knew there were two kinds of kids: those who got Flintstones vitamins and those who didn't. Now, years later, there are still conflicting ideas about whether we really need to supplement our diets with extra vitamins. No one disagrees that it is safe to take the RDI (reference daily intake) amounts. But for people with liver disease, it is probably not a good idea to exceed what used to be called our RDA, or recommended daily allowance. And we should definitely avoid extra iron.

In a nutshell, vitamins are either fat-soluble or water-soluble. Vitamins A, D, E, and K are fat soluble, which means they don't dissolve in water and are stored by fat in your body. The other vitamins (eight B vitamins and vitamin C) are water-soluble and can easily dissolve in—and be passed through and out of—your body. Thirteen different types of vitamins and 22 minerals are required by your body in order to function.

Vitamins aren't all created equal, however. Some, called antioxidants, carry out more critical tasks, such as reducing your risk of heart disease or cancer and boosting your immune system. These antioxidants help our body get rid of harmful atoms called free radicals that circulate in your system, damaging healthy cells and tissues. HBV may cause us to have more of these free radicals in our bodies. Vitamins C, E, and beta-carotene have also been shown to help your body fight them off, and those with HBV should be sure to get plenty of antioxidants either in our diets or supplements or both. It's best to get as many as you can in your diet. Scientists say that it's not just about getting the right vitamin; it's about how this vitamin interacts with other nutrients. Discuss the particulars of your diet with your doctor and discuss whether she thinks you need to take extra vitamins.

The following vitamins are particularly helpful to the liver in normal doses:

- ◯ B Complex
- ◯ Vitamin E
- ◯ Vitamin C
- ◯ Vitamin K
- ◯ Folic acid

Vitamin E also acts as an antioxidant in the body and helps maintain levels of **glutathione**, which is particularly important for people with hepatitis. Although the federal dietary guidelines suggest getting 400 milligrams per day, it may be the most difficult vitamin for us to get from our diet. Many of those I interviewed take 100 to 400 milligrams per day in vitamin form.

Don't overdo it with vitamins

However, since A, D, E and K are also fat-soluble, you don't want to take large supplements of these, as too much of a good thing is detrimental to your health. Vitamin C, for example, increases iron absorption, so you should avoid large doses of it. Some doctors recommend children's vitamins for people with HBV, as long as they don't contain iron.

Avoid too much iron and vitamin A

In particular, excess iron in your diet can be toxic. Your liver is the natural repository of iron in your body, and it plays an essential role in regulating blood iron levels and synthesizing transferritin (an iron-binding protein) and ferritin, which is the major iron storage protein. Inflammation of the liver can interrupt these processes, releasing too much iron into the system and also causing hepatocytes to store too much of it.

Avoid iron supplements and check food labels for added iron. For example, some breakfast cereals can have dangerous levels of added iron. Some iron is important, particularly for those with anemia or menstruating women. Moderation is the key here.

Vitamin A can also be toxic to the liver. Beta-carotene or foods rich in vitamin A are a better choice, meaning that you can feel free to drink carrot juice, but should avoid supplements and foods with added vitamin A.

Some minerals are especially important for your liver

- ◯ Selenium
- ◯ Zinc
- ◯ Calcium
- ◯ Chromium
- ◯ Copper

Antioxidants and supplements

Lipoic Acid is a potent antioxidant and one of the best liver detoxifiers. It's found in tiny amounts in some foods like spinach, beef, and potatoes. Some people take 100 mg-supplement a day with food.

Glutathione is an amino acid and has an important role in the body's antioxidant defense system. It's required for a variety of metabolic processes. Among the foods that contain glutathione are avocados, asparagus, grapefruit, potatoes, acorn squash, tomatoes, broccoli, oranges, strawberries, peaches, zucchini, and spinach. **Limonene** is a phytochemical and boosts a glutathione-containing enzyme that has antioxidant properties and helps to detoxify chemicals, thus protecting the liver. It is found in cherries, citrus fruit peels, celery, fennel, soy, and wheat. Glutathione isn't that well absorbed by the body, so not every doctor recommends supplements.

Coenzyme Q-10 (CoQ-10) is becoming a popular supplement, since it is said to help prevent cardiovascular or gum disease and support the immune system. It may also boost the effect of vitamin E. CoQ-10 is actually manufactured by our bodies in small, but not significant, amounts.

IN A SENTENCE:

> *Your mother was right—it's important to know about the basics of good nutrition, especially when you have hepatitis.*

learning

Other HBV Symptoms

IN DAY 7 we learned about fatigue, the most common symptom of HBV. There are, unfortunately, other symptoms, but in order to avoid blaming hepatitis B for all our aches and pains, we need to familiarize ourselves with the most common. If you have liver scarring and are experiencing symptoms, you know that they seem to come in waves. And just when you think you've resolved one, another presents itself. As mentioned before, those who have more severe liver damage will be more likely to experience the following most common symptoms.

Liver pain or discomfort is disconcerting but not uncommon

Some of us experience daily general discomfort in our right upper quadrant. Others experience sharp pains when they twist their abdomen or lean over. We all seem to have some kind of sensation from our livers. And we refer to this as liver pain, despite the fact the liver doesn't experience pain. The membrane around the liver does have nerve endings however, as do the surrounding organs.

People with HBV sometimes have joint pain

You may think you have a touch of arthritis or **arthralgia**. However, joint stiffness and pain, along with other side effects that do not have their genesis specifically in the liver, are called extra-hepatic manifestations of HBV. This means that HBV literally manifests itself outside of the liver. You may feel either stiffness or aches in your shoulder, hips, knees, or other joints. It is believed that hepatitis viruses may also lead to fibromyalgia, or pain in connective tissues, muscles, and joint with or without fatigue. Ask your doctor what she recommends for your joint pain. Since it may be unwise to take too many pain relievers, you may want to use heat therapy (shower, sauna, bath, or heating pad) instead of medication. Sometimes a reduction in viral load can lessen joint pain, and your joint pain may come in intervals.

HBV can bring on bloating, irritable bowel episodes, and diarrhea

Bloating, gas, and rumbling stomachs and intestines can be common if you have HBV. It can lead to embarrassing moments in meetings with clients or at school. And stress may exacerbate all of these symptoms. Don't eat fat on an empty stomach and avoid saturated and trans fats and red meat. Eating smaller meals more frequently throughout the day can help minimize this discomfort, as well as limiting caffeine, dairy products, and fatty or spicy foods. Stay hydrated. Keep track of how long these symptoms last, and call your doctor if they do not get better after you've modified your diet.

Light or clay-colored stools are a sign of what's happening in your liver

Call your doctor if you notice very dark, tarry stools, as this may mean that bleeding is occurring somewhere in your digestive tract. Clay-colored stools are not unusual to see in people who have HBV and cirrhosis, and may point to an obstruction of bile flow from the liver or a lack of bile salt production. Unfortunately, you may have noticed that your stools are quite odorous, reeking of sulfur.

Thin strands of stool for extended periods or unusually light or very dark stools should also be reported to your doctor. See Month 3 for more information about stools.

Varicose and spider veins
are sometimes visible in people with liver damage

Severe fibrosis or cirrhosis can sometimes cause dilated veins on the skin's surface that are visible to the eye. Also known as varicose veins, they develop when blood from the intestines has a hard time getting back to the heart through the portal vein due to liver scarring. The blood tries to find short cuts and goes back through other channels called tributaries. These veins can also develop due to other conditions, such as obesity.

Spider nevi or spider telangiectasias are fine veins that sometimes appear on our noses, nostrils, or cheeks. These are usually found above the nipple line. One identifying aspect is that they "blanch" or disappear when slight pressure is applied to them. "Spiders," like varicose veins, are due to portal hypertension (PHT) and cirrhosis. They are like arterial micro-aneurysms under the skin, possibly arising from the effect of increased estrogen in the body due to its prolonged degradation by an injured liver. They occur in roughly 10 percent of people with chronic HBV without cirrhosis, so theoretically it is possible for some of us to have them without severe damage. Pregnant women and those with rheumatoid arthritis are also susceptible. Although spider veins can be due to HBV, they are also just part of getting older.

You may experience night sweats

Waking up in the middle of the night and finding your sheets soaked can be a distressing thing. We call these episodes night sweats, and they seem to occur more frequently in people with elevated enzymes and high viral loads, though the exact relationship is not clear and isn't well documented in medical literature. It is quite possible that your primary physician may doubt these episodes are HBV related, especially if you are female and nearing menopause. Many people I've interviewed—men and women—have experienced them. If they continue for long periods and are coupled with fatigue or joint pain, you may be experiencing a flare-up of your HBV.

Some people have rashes, itching, and dryness

A good number of people are led to a correct diagnosis of HBV through initial complaints about itching to their doctors. Itching, also known as

pruritus, is one of the most common and perhaps one of the more annoying symptoms that many of us have to deal with. Among other things, it is caused by a buildup of toxins in your blood. Dryness and scaling may also accompany your itching. Your doctor may prescribe a mild topical steroid cream to soothe your itching. Others suggest taking vitamin K supplements or using topical oatmeal-based or natural creams. I find that even a once-over with a brand-name skin cream such as Aveeno, Cetaphil, or Lubriderm does the trick, especially after a shower, though only if applied before my skin dries. Avoid sudden temperature changes like stepping out of the sauna into a cold shower. This can cause itching that is entirely unrelated to HBV.

Gianotti-Crosti syndrome sounds like some new delicious pasta dish. Too bad it actually refers to a form of dermatitis that shows up on legs, buttocks, neck, and face. It looks just like a rash or acne, with red, raised bumps that seem to contain pus but do not. It is often associated with children with HBV or other diseases, but can also appear in adults. Fortunately it usually doesn't itch. The spots are very small in diameter and are deep red or even purple, due to broken blood capillaries. I had Gianotti-Crosti on my upper legs and buttocks at intervals for many years, despite the fact that long-term presence is fairly rare. To me the skin irritation looked like acne or very large goose bumps. When I changed my diet and stopped smoking, it disappeared entirely.

Lichen Planus sometimes occurs in those with HCV, but can show up in anyone with liver disease. It is also induced by stress or contact with chemicals. While it often chooses to appear on your wrists or ankles, lichen planus can also show up in your mouth or on your tongue or nails.

Some people say that their skin is particularly sensitive to scrapes, scratching, or repetitive friction. I've had minor bleeding after lightly scratching or rubbing an area on my arms or legs, while others have mentioned similar episodes occurring during or after sex.

IN A SENTENCE:

> *You may be fortunate not to experience any of them, but HBV can potentially cause a wide range of symptoms.*

Avoiding Toxic
People, Places, and Things

TAKING CARE of your body naturally entails not just changing your diet and exercising, but also changing or altering your environment. This is typical advice for those with alcohol or chemical dependencies. You can't just go off to a 28-day program without changing the environment while you're gone. You have to treat the environment while you treat the disease by altering and adapting your home, work, and social settings. The same idea applies to life with HBV.

Making change happen in real life is tough because it involves your friends, family, and colleagues, not to mention your most entrenched ideas about happiness. These are the basic building blocks of life, and constructing a new life platform in which you find new pleasures and pursuits is difficult and doesn't happen overnight.

For example, I have a friend with hepatitis C who owns a bar and restaurant. The business has been in his family for generations, and it is a beautiful and entertaining place. But try as he may, he's unable to break free of his smoking and drinking habits. His health, of course, is getting worse as the years go by. His entire bar staff smokes and patrons buy rounds of drinks for my friend and his staff. He has no resistance, and is torn between the love of his business and his love of his liver.

We've spoken a few times about what it's going to take to get him to change, and have discussed every possible scenario: hire someone else to run the business, change the nature of the business (to a vegetarian restaurant!), or sell this particular business and start another, such as a bakery or home delivery service. I'm afraid that he's not ready enough yet to choose any of these options. At the moment, he's procrastinating, hoping his liver will hold out.

How you choose to make life changes happen is, of course, entirely up to you. You will also have to gauge how important it is to safeguard your health and how important it is to safeguard your social life. The key is to first examine all the situations you find yourself in that are not liver-friendly. Then, write a list of possible alternatives that get you excited. If you spend every Friday night in the pub with your colleagues, find an activity that you'd be excited about doing instead, like a drawing class, French lessons, or skydiving. Counterbalance the prospect of potentially losing old acquaintances with the probability that you'll meet new friends with similar nontoxic interests.

You may want to start avoiding toxic people

You may have never realized that you had toxic people around you until HBV entered your life. Many of the people I've interviewed talk about how having hepatitis has deeply affected their relationships in a *positive* way. Many of us have found more satisfying and profound friendships since our diagnosis, and I truly love hearing these stories. It would seem that there really is a silver lining to our suffering.

But to get there, we often have to start eliminating the negative or toxic people in our lives, whether they be friends, colleagues, or casual acquaintances. What do we mean by toxic? Toxic can be literal—those that drink or smoke too much or drag you to fast food joints—but it can also be figurative—the people who say negative things or add stress to your day.

Draw three columns on a piece of paper. Write "Positive," "Neutral," and "Negative" at the top of each column. Then put the names of everyone you know in the columns. This will seem cold and calculated. It is. But it is meant as an exercise only. After you have written the names, take the names in the negative column and write what it will take to salvage your friendship or connection to this person. If the person is always bossing you around or critical of you, you can either avoid them or ask them to adapt their behavior.

Toxic people are as harmful to our bodies and minds as other toxins. They increase our stress level, diminish our morale, and make life hellish. If they are abusive, don't argue with them. Remain calm and don't interrupt. Try to take a deep breath and simply state how you feel. If the situation deteriorates and the person becomes irate or insulting, simply turn on your heel and walk away. If you find that the person still stresses you out after thirty minutes, go to a private place and talk out loud to yourself. It may sound silly but it is effective. Say to yourself, "I will not let this person harm me. I refuse to let them harm me." Take deep breaths and continue repeating as necessary.

What if I'm the negative person?

Of course, you have a little problem if everyone thinks *you're* the toxic one. And they may, especially if they think that you've become bitter because of HBV. If you have this virus, you know full well that resisting victimization or giving in to self-pity is tough, as there are so many good opportunities. Being negative is part of the natural journey to acceptance, but we shouldn't get stuck in negativity.

Avoid everyday toxins

Most of us use a good number of the following products every day. You should not feel so alarmed that you run out and throw all of the following things into a Dumpster. However, it is a good idea to eliminate as many as you can, using the phase-out schedule. Almost all of the following products are available in nontoxic, ecofriendly versions.

Cleaning solutions: These solutions can contain alcohol, isopropyl alcohol, sodium hydroxide, and other chemicals that enter your systems as fumes and are toxic to your liver. Try buying nontoxic, ecofriendly cleaning supplies, or just use a vinegar and water solution. I recommend using Natural Wonder, a glass and multisurface cleaner made by EnviroSmart Products, a Chicago-based company. It contains only corn, coconut, and citrus derived cleaners, and is just as effective as any other glass cleaner. I made my office start using it because I would have to leave the room when people used strong chemical cleaners on dry-erase boards. Your local health food store or organic grocery probably has a range of liver-friendly products.

Toiletries: Try to avoid chemical-based products like nail polish, hair spray, foot sprays, deodorants, and perfumes, particularly those with aerosol sprays. Natural equivalents are readily available if you look for them. Also, read the labels on these products. It's probably a good idea to avoid any cosmetic product that is full of chemicals and chemical dyes such as diethanolamine, monoethanolamine, triethanolamine, imidazolidinyl, polyethylene glycol, propylene glycol, and sodium lauryl sulfate. No need to be alarmist here, but if your liver is slow to eliminate toxins, we don't need any more chemicals in and on our bodies than absolutely necessary.

Yard supplies: Fertilizers, gas, plant sprays, bug sprays, pool chlorine, et cetera are harmful to your liver. I don't use weed killer on my lawn, and at least those who have HBV-infected children would be wise not to use chemical fertilizers or weed killers. This is a great opportunity to let someone else clean the pool and do your yard work for you.

Household paints and art supplies: Oil paints, paint thinners, paint strippers, spray paints, epoxies, and other solvents should be avoided, as well as permanent markers and glues. If you paint with oils you should think about doing it outside, or switch to watercolors or acrylics. Buy and wear a respirator for unavoidable jobs.

If your work involves frequent use of chemicals and solvents or exposes you to exhaust fumes, you may want to think about finding a less toxic environment. If you do come into contact with these above-mentioned substances by accident, have a shower, drink plenty of filtered water, and treat yourself to a nice sauna.

Electronic equipment: Avoid electric blankets, and if you have an electric alarm clock don't keep it next to your head. They generate large electrical fields and may interfere with healing. Use a hands-free headset when using your cell phone.

Smoke and exhaust: Cigarette smoke contains benzopyrene, cyanide, acetaldehyde, tars, and dozens of other toxins. Avoid fuel exhaust (even gas lawnmowers or generators).

Saunas give your liver a break

Saunas have been used since ancient times as a natural, noninvasive method for removing toxins from the body. They can also be relaxing and fun. Get that image of those gray-haired men in togas or sexy Finns out of your mind now, because saunas can help your skin carry out some of the detoxing tasks for which your liver is usually responsible.

There are seemingly a billion man-made chemicals that we come into contact with everyday—from food, air, water, and household cleaning supplies. Most of these environmental toxins are fat-soluble, so they naturally gravitate to the lipids or fatty tissues in our bodies.

Our livers take on the brunt of the task of removing these toxins by making them water-soluble so that the body can help to excrete them. A sauna can streamline this process by convincing these chemicals to come out of hiding and get into the body's general circulation. And if elevated heat can convince toxins to come out, who's to say that HBV can't be coaxed out of our nooks and crannies, too? In fact, studies have shown that the therapeutic use of saunas can lower liver enzymes and decrease glucose and cholesterol levels. They also give you an all-over glow.

While you're in the sauna, the temperature of your body's surface gradually increases, causing your blood vessels to dilate and circulation in the skin to increase. Your blood pressure slowly but surely goes down while your heartbeat increases to maintain normal blood pressure. That's why we may feel faint if we stay in the sauna too long. It's best to start very slow—just a few minutes at a lower temperature, then slowly work your way up to longer sessions and slightly higher temperatures.

Set the temperature gauge quite low, because you want to sweat, not cook. Some say that in order for you to sweat enough to make a difference, the temperature must be low enough that you don't lose too much water or electrolytes. You don't have to buy a boar-bristle brush, but you do need to make sure that you carefully wash all of your oily sweat off your body afterwards. Drink plenty of filtered water beforehand, and continue drinking water during and after. I prefer the dry saunas to Turkish baths (steam saunas) because I can put my feet up and read the entire *New York Times* without it turning into mush in my hands. But either will help you remove toxins from your body.

Afterwards, I feel like I don't have HBV for at least three hours. I think more clearly, have more energy, fewer colds and bouts of flu, and I sleep much better.

Hopefully your local gym, Y, or swimming pool will have either a Turkish bath or sauna. New freestanding personal models are also available if you like your privacy and have a little extra room in your bathroom and a little extra cash in your wallet. Pregnant women and people with low blood pressure should avoid taking saunas, and you should consult with your doctor before trying it for yourself.

IN A SENTENCE:

> *It is wise to avoid as many toxins—chemical or otherwise—as you can, whether they are in your air, water, food, or in the company you keep.*

learning

Which Treatment is Right for You?

You will be helping to choose which treatment is right for you

KNOWING WHICH treatment to choose is not an easy thing. And unlike other diseases, there are a lot of gray areas when it comes to treating HBV. Not only do you have to decide whether to treat or not, you also have to decide which treatment or which combination of treatments, and whether to start combination treatments concurrently or staggered. Since many variables come into play and many new medications are on the horizon, it is a good idea for you to take an active role in deciding which treatment strategy is right for you. This will take considerable brainpower and patience.

Most hepatologists agree that hepatitis is not a one-drug disease. Unfortunately, the FDA has not yet approved combination therapies for use against HBV. The more you learn about HBV treatment, the more you realize that we are all on the cutting edge. We are the guinea pigs. This means that not only does your doctor not have all the answers, but also that you will be taking more responsibility for your own treatment and keeping abreast of the latest treatments. It is important to stay informed, especially if you are letting your primary physician care for your HBV rather than a specialist. You will very likely know just as much as your doctor and will have to rely on your intuition just as much as he will.

The great challenge of HBV treatment is not just to seroconvert, but also to stay that way without having the virus build up resistance to the drug by slightly altering its structure. We call this mutating, but I find that this term conjures fear. Some think that this mutant virus is less harmful than the original, or "wild-type," virus. I will return to this discussion later when we talk about **Lamivudine**, another possible treatment for HBV. In short, we aim to seroconvert and keep our viral load as low as possible.

Interferon vs. Lamivudine

While both Interferon and Lamivudine are effective treatments, they don't work for everyone. The following is a table of information that may assist you in differentiating between these two main treatments.

	Interferon	**Lamivudine**
Year Approved by FDA	1991	1998
Company	Schering-Plough	GlaxoSmithKline
Website	www.schering.com	www.gsk.com
Mechanism	Immunomodulator– Mimics immune system's infection fighting response	Nucleoside Analogue– Interrupts manufacture of enzyme needed for viral reproduction
Side Effects	Yes Flu-like symptoms, loss of appetite, depression, hair loss, lowering of blood counts	Minimal; occasional muscle pain or headaches
Dosage	Injections 1–3 times per week	Oral pill Usually 1 per day

	Interferon	Lamivudine
Length of Treatment	4 to 6 months	1 year or more
Virus develops resistance/mutation?	No	Yes. Mutation occurs in 50% after 3 years of use
Success rate of therapy: e antigen and HBV/DNA loss	30–40%	30–33%
Loss of HBsAg	In 1–10% of those who also lose HBeAg	Rare
Recommended pretreatment enzymes levels	2–5 times high range of ALT and AST	2–5 times high range of ALT and AST
Recommended pretreatment HBV DNA levels	Low	Low
Use for precore mutant (more common in Asians) with e antigen negative?	No (Has been used in the presence of abnormal liver enzymes)	Yes
Use for Fibrosis?	Yes	Yes
Use for Cirrhosis?	Limited	Yes, even in those with decompensation
Does it improve liver histology? (condition)	Yes but only in those with e antigen loss	Improves even if e antigen is not lost
Use for children?	Yes	Yes

Different approaches

INTERFERON

What is Interferon?

Interferon got its name because it interferes with a virus's ability to replicate. It can protect healthy cells from being invaded by HBV. Interferon is also produced naturally, and is secreted by our body's cells to fight off viral, bacterial, and parasitic infections. Once secreted, it binds itself to cell membranes and carries out a number of complex tasks that are difficult to pronounce, let alone understand. In short, however, Interferon reduces viral replication and helps to minimize liver inflammation by doing the following:

○ Eliminates cells infected by HBV by recruiting secret agents that are already present in the body. One of these agents is a set of proteins that get released on the cell's surface, blocking the entry of the virus. The other agent trains our own killer T cells to recognize and kill infected cells.
○ Enhances its own talent for destroying the virus and learns to stop the viral sweatshop in the liver cells.

Given that Interferon can also slow cell division, it is sometimes used to put the brakes on cancer cell proliferation. If treatment is successful, it can help return HBV to its dormant stage and postpone the onset of cirrhosis and the likelihood of liver cancer.

Alpha Interferon is a synthetic version of our body's own naturally produced interferon. There are a few different brands: Intron A, Roferon, and Infergen. There are new versions just coming out onto the market, which reduce the number of injections necessary to complete treatment, because the Interferon is suspended in polyethylene glycol (PEG), a gellike substance that offers a timed release of Interferon into your system. This reduces the number of injections from daily or three per week to only one. Many people report that they have fewer side effects with this new **pegylated Interferon**.

Interferon isn't for everyone

There are many important considerations you will have to make along with your doctor before choosing Interferon, and you should take an active role in deciding whether you want to take the injections or not. You may not qualify if you:

○ Are pregnant
○ Suffer from heart or kidney disease
○ Have thyroid imbalances or anemia
○ Have a transplanted liver
○ Lack a sufficient support system or suffer from mental illness
○ Have cirrhosis

Interferon is the ideal drug for some people

There are, however, indicators that make you a better candidate for Interferon treatment, which are considered reliable after years of research about the effect of Interferon on HBV. The following is a list of indicators that mean you are more likely to respond to Interferon:

○ Recent biopsy which shows moderate to severe inflammation
○ Elevated ALT and AST for more than six months (2 to 5 times normal)
○ DNA in the mid to low range (less than 200 pg /ml)
○ Recent infection
○ e antigen positive
○ Absence of other serious health condition
○ HIV negative status
○ No ascites, varices, or encephalopathy
○ Non Asian lineage (since Asians generally have normal ALT and high HBV DNA)

Your blood tests should also be within normal range to qualify for (and continue taking) Interferon:

○ Albumin
○ Bilirubin
○ Hemoglobin
○ Platelet count
○ Prothrombin time
○ White cell counts

There are other considerations that could rule out the use of Interferon:

○ White blood cell count lower than 3,000
○ Blood hemoglobin under 10 grams per deciliter
○ Platelets lower than 50,000
○ The presence of severe cirrhosis with complications like decreased liver function, ascites, encephalopathy, bleeding from varices
○ Clinically significant depression or lack of family support
○ Active drug or alcohol abuse

You may experience side effects, but you can take steps to alleviate them

Interferon side effects tend to appear most prominently in the first few weeks. You may want to schedule time off for a week or two to coincide with the start of the course of treatment. Some suffer from thinning hair or even significant hair loss (it will grow back after treatment), and you may experience headaches, chills, fever, or night sweats. Interferon may also leave you with a metallic taste in your mouth, which you can minimize with frequent brushing, mouthwash, or gum. Sometimes you may even experience a flare of symptoms or enzymes on treatment. This is often a good thing because it means that your body is responding to the Interferon. Here are some of the most common side effects.

Flu-like symptoms: Drinking plenty of fluids before and after your injection will help minimize Interferon's side effects. If you have significant discomfort after the shot, try taking the injection just before going to bed so you can sleep through the worst symptoms. Your doctor may allow you to take Tylenol® or Aspirin-Free Excedrin® on occasion if you feel you need it, but not NSAIDs.

Loss of appetite: It is tough to work up an appetite when you're not at all sure that you can keep your food down. Try eating small meals or healthy snacks throughout the day instead of large meals. Some drink Gatorade for energy, and clear juices can help provide energy and nourishment. A few people I've interviewed have found that marijuana or marinol pills stimulate their appetite, but somehow it seems counterproductive to introduce more toxins (particularly those of uncontrolled and unknown origin) into your body.

Nausea: Avoid food smells that bother you. Ask your doctor what she prefers in terms of over-the-counter medications. Try drinking ginger or chamomile tea.

Fatigue: As mentioned before, keep a regular sleep schedule and get at least eight hours every night. If you are still working, ask for reasonable accommodation, such as a late start the day of your injection or shorter hours. Walking or light exercise will help mitigate some of your fatigue.

Depression: Make sure you have a support system in place before you start treatment. Do your homework and find a suitable therapist before starting treatment. It may be easier to make this important decision before you find yourself in the thick of treatment. Ask for a free introductory visit so that the therapist has an idea of what you're like before treatment. Let your best friends know that depression is a possible side effect before you start treatment so they can be aware and more objective about any changes they perceive in your mood or behavior. Some changes you might experience include sleeping longer than usual, eating too much or too little, low self-esteem, agitation or nervousness, lack of concentration, and negative thoughts. Keep track of your moods and let your doctor know if you feel that any or all of these are becoming unmanageable.

If depression continues, you may need to discuss taking a medication to help control it. This may mean a prescription for Zoloft or Prozac, for example. Most doctors say that these medications do not harm the liver, but if you decide to take them you will need to be vigilant and attentive to any side effects that you may experience, physically and mentally.

Other possible side effects: Very few people (less than 5 percent) experience thyroid abnormalities. A few may notice changes in their eyes. If you have diabetes, high blood pressure, or have preexisting eye conditions, be sure to let your doctor know. A few people have experienced restless nights or vivid nightmares.

You will probably be taught how to give yourself injections

If you don't know anyone in your immediate family who is able to give you injections, you will need to be trained to do so. Interferon injections are usually given subcutaneously like insulin shots, just under the skin. They are not intramuscular injections, that is, deep into the muscle tissue. You will want to inject yourself by alternating sites (i.e., left thigh one day, right thigh the next), and it will help to drink plenty of filtered water or noncaffeinated drinks before and after the injection. Taking the injections an hour before bedtime may help you sleep through the initial side effects.

You may not respond to Interferon treatment

If you decide to try Interferon, you will be tested every 1 to 3 months to see if your body is responding. Your doctor will look at your ALT and AST levels, your HBV DNA, and e antigen. Specifically, your doctor will want to see if you have lost HBeAg and developed the e antibody.

You will be classified as a "complete" or "sustained responder," a "partial responder," or a "non-responder." Unfortunately, over 60 percent of those with HBV who try Interferon have no response whatsoever.

You may relapse after Interferon treatment

Five to ten percent of those who do respond completely to treatment will relapse within six to twelve months from the end of treatment. Even though you may initially respond to treatment with Interferon, there is a chance that once you stop treatment that you can relapse, though this is uncommon. Relapse rates are higher in those who are e antigen negative to begin with.

Remember that there are promising treatments on the horizon

Doctors sometimes get so excited about new drugs that are currently being tested in human studies that they start to sound like stockbrokers.

"Time to run out and buy some Fill-in-the-blank stock," is a common way of expressing excitement about positive findings of reduced viral load or overall energy levels. In Month 6 you will find an in-depth discussion of the drugs that are currently in Phase III trials and have successfully jumped through the first two FDA hoops.

LAMIVUDINE

Lamivudine, also known as Epivir, 3TC, Heptovir, or abroad as Zeffix, is a nucleoside analogue and was initially introduced as a treatment against HIV. It was approved for treatment of HBV in 1998. Given that it seems to work well for a wide range of people (including those with cirrhosis and transplant recipients), it has quickly become the leading treatment for chronic hepatitis B. In fact, almost everyone who takes Lamivudine sees a rapid decrease in HBV DNA over a very short time. The good news is that a rapid decrease in DNA means our livers may experience less inflammation and, subsequently, less scarring.

Although Lamivudine is very effective in quickly reducing viral load, it can't penetrate the nucleus of our liver cells. This means that it can't get to the part of the virus (called cccDNA) that was previously able to penetrate the cells. It reduces replication because it robs the spare parts that float outside of the liver cell of oxygen, inhibiting them from producing other spare parts.

In effect, Lamivudine stops all the hens (complete viruses) but lets the HBV eggs stay warm and safe inside the host nuclei. Both the virus and Lamivudine play a game of chicken in which whomever quits first loses. Unfortunately, HBV is so warm and happy in the hepatocyte that it doesn't feel the need to leave its cocoon. Some doctors say we'll have a more effective drug out on the market soon that will take care of this egg. Unfortunately we just haven't seen it yet, though a drug currently in Phase III trials called **Entecavir** shows that promise.

Lamivudine isn't for everyone. If you already have low ALT, Lamivudine—like Interferon—may not work for you. Steve Bingham's metaphor for this phenomenon is memorable: "you have to wait until the gopher (virus) becomes active and sticks his head out of his hole (in this case the liver cell) before you whack him with a shovel (Lamivudine)."

Lamivudine may also help improve your energy levels. It is not uncommon to experience a boost of energy after a few weeks of taking Lamivudine. This is due to the fact that your liver is finally getting a break from the virus. My viral load dropped from 5.7 million copies/ml to 200 copies/ml in less than six months. I hadn't felt that energetic since high school. Others say that Lamivudine helps them have regular bowel movements and less bloating.

Lamivudine has very few side effects, if any

The recommended dose of Lamivudine for hepatitis B is once daily, orally, at 100mg. If a person is co-infected with HIV this dosage may be twice daily at 150mg. It is very well-tolerated with minimal side effects. Some people, myself included, experience mild, throbbing headaches. I've not been able to find others who have experienced other side effects, but that could be because if they exist they mimic the most common HBV complaints such as diarrhea, nausea, skin rash, abdominal pain, coughing, and muscle aches.

If you stop taking Lamivudine, you may experience a flare

Lamivudine does a remarkable job of lowering your viral load within weeks of taking it. However, if you stop treatment, the virus can quickly replicate, possibly causing a flare. Some doctors suggest slowly weaning off Lamivudine; others suggest continuing to take it even if your viral load entirely disappears. If you do decide to stop, you should monitor your viral load carefully, and have a contingency plan ready in case it does.

Lamivudine isn't perfect, but it buys time

One hitch with Lamivudine is that our bodies may develop resistance to Lamivudine over time. Lamivudine monotherapy leads to resistance within 2 years in roughly 30 percent of those who take it. Your chance of developing resistance increases the longer you take it, jumping up to 50 percent after three years and 90 percent after four years. See Month 4 for a more thorough discussion of how viruses can develop resistance to Lamivudine.

Since Lamivudine is so affordable, doesn't require injections, and has few, if any side effects, it is easy to see why so many choose it. Many of us choose to take it for the time being in the hopes that something better will be offered either alone or in combination with it. We're anxiously awaiting FDA approval of another drug that may be combined in a kind of drug cocktail, much like new drug combinations used for HIV. As mentioned above, see Month 7 for a more in depth discussion of what you may be taking in a few months or years.

IN A SENTENCE:

There are many considerations to make before choosing a treatment strategy, and you should talk with your doctor to make the best decision for you.

Exercise

HBV LOVES a couch potato. So you'll want to do what you can to overcome your resistance to exercise and get in gear. Starting an exercise program is like jumping into a cold lake— you know it'll eventually feel good, but you fear the shock to your system. It's much easier to just watch the others enjoy themselves. If you're still stuck on the sidelines, you've probably forgotten what a rush you get from the endorphins your body sends to your brain as a reward for your efforts. Like drugs, endorphins are addictive. They have a chemical structure that is similar to morphine and they naturally relieve pain.

You simply need to gain a little momentum in the first few weeks for your body to build up this healthy dependency.

Exercise is treatment

Here's a mental trick to help you move your butt. A slight semantic shift may help you adapt your thinking about exercise: simply think of it as *physical therapy* that's *detoxing your liver*. With this subtle mental shift, you can overcome years of built-up resentment towards all those jocks in high school. Exercise, along with diet, is very effective treatment. To get there you can use a kind of phase-in system that is the inversion of your HBV diet phase-out period.

If you're exercising you're probably losing weight, and if you lose weight you probably will feel better about yourself, and if you feel better about yourself, your level of self-esteem will augment other life areas.

Karin K. is a champion speed skater despite having stage 3 fibrosis. She is convinced that exercise has helped her minimize the effects of HBV, both mentally and physically: "Competing against 'healthy' people makes you feel much better about having a chronic illness. Intense physical activity leaves little room for the mind to wander or worry, and it is a time that I rarely think about any of my troubles. I see it as a form of meditation for people (like me) who are not good enough at sitting still to meditate in more traditional ways. I think that intense exercise is a good natural pain killer too, without side effects. You have a reason to eat and rest well, keep a journal of what you are doing and how it makes you feel, and you avoid doing unhealthy things because they might interfere with performance."

To get your body ready for the HBV phase-in exercise program, you should have a look at these pages and discuss them with your doctor. Every knee, lung, and pulse is different, and you don't want to exacerbate any other conditions you might have.

You don't have to break world records

You don't have to push too hard—no one is standing over you with a stopwatch. If you are older or confined to a bed or wheelchair, it is still possible to exercise. Ask a physical therapist to help you find movements that won't hurt you. The essential thing at the beginning is that every day you do just a little bit more than you did the day before. You should aim for a target of at least 30 minutes of exercise every day. Joining a class at the Y or gym is a good way to get started. If you prefer to stay in the privacy of your own home, try videos or exercise books. *Yoga for Wimps: Poses for the Flexibly Impaired* (Sterling, 2000) for example, is a good beginner's book.

Many people find that it makes sense to join a gym as close to work as possible. That way you can eat the low-fat lunch you brought from home at your desk and use your lunch break for the treadmill and your favorite soap on the gym's TV monitors. You can also sneak in a short sauna. Try taking a five-minute sauna *before* your workout—it will warm up your muscles and allow your body to be more flexible when you do your stretching exercises.

If you've never belonged to a gym before, set appointments with a few of them and take a tour. Most gyms even allow you to have a free workout after your tour. Look at the courses offered and how often they are offered. Ask the gym about their low-impact classes, such as yoga or beginning

Pilates method. Ask other people around you how they like the gym, and make sure that the gym offers saunas and massages. Most gyms include a few sessions with a personal trainer to acquaint you with the gym and its equipment. You may even want to purchase a block of sessions, as gyms offer volume discounts on personal trainers. Ask the gym if any of the trainers have experience in working with people who have chronic illnesses. I did and found it to be immensely helpful because I learned how to keep my heart rate low and stay within the fat-burning range. I also learned to isolate my muscle groups and concentrate on one (e.g., shoulders, arms, chest, legs) every day in order to let muscles rest for a few days between workouts.

If you just can't bear the thought of joining a gym, you can still be creative. Try parking a little farther from the store at the mall or walk up stairs instead of taking the elevator. Ask a friend to go for a walk in a park—nothing makes exercise more fun than having a friend with you. And yes, vigorous house cleaning (with nontoxic, ecofriendly cleaning products) will count towards your daily half hour.

Start breathing

Once you've gotten a go-ahead from your doctor, start with a baby step: breathe. You don't need drugs to get high. All you need is a bit of oxygen and your lungs. And breathing doesn't really take an extra energy on your part. For example you can take a few minutes at bedtime or upon waking for deep breathing exercises.

Try this (sitting, standing, or laying down): put one hand on your lower stomach (your belt line) and the other just above your breastbone. Take a very deep breath. Which hand rises up when you breathe? Probably the hand on your breastbone. Now try again, attempting to get air to your lower abdomen. You should now feel your stomach push out more. We tend to keep our abdominal muscles tightened (to look svelte at the supermarket) but while doing these exercises, your goal is to take in oxygen and help your liver, not to win a beauty pageant.

Try this for a few minutes at first and then work up to periods of 10–15 minutes or more. You may feel slightly light-headed, but you will also feel quite refreshed and relaxed. If you're sitting, try combining these breathing exercises with light exercises such as rolling your shoulders or slow neck bends.

While doing these exercises, I keep my hands over my right rib cage and imagine that this oxygen is going straight to my liver. The combination of my hands' warmth and deep breathing does wonders for me, especially when I have mild brain fog or fatigue. And it doesn't cost a thing. If you find that these breathing exercises really work for you, you may want to take it to the next step and take a meditation or yoga class.

Try Tai Chi

Tai Chi, also referred to as Qi Gong or Chi Kung, originated in ancient China. Not surprisingly, it originated as a medical practice, but over the centuries, has slowly developed into a spiritual practice and martial art. It offers two winning and simple ingredients: graceful movement and breathing. Tai Chi is gradually becoming popular in the United States. It is low-intensity/low-impact and has an unhurried and elegant air about it. Despite its appearance it can increase strength and balance, enhance range of motion, and improve your coordination and posture. Clinical trials have shown that it can reduce your blood pressure and heart rate.

Tai Chi consists of a series of poetically named movements that encourage continuous motion. It can be performed anywhere at any time. What I like about Tai Chi is that it can help me feel like I'm slowing down my mind and my life. Like meditation, it helps me savor time. Although doing the same movements over and over may seem boring at first, with time and practice, it will become more challenging. While it's easy to learn basic Tai Chi movements, mastery can take a lifetime. Tai Chi is about learning to be introspective—recognizing the stress in your body, and then releasing it. You probably won't work up a sweat, but you will very likely feel invigorated and refreshed. And who can resist a movement called "Wind Rolls the Lotus Leaves"?

Start with low-impact activities like walking, swimming, or yoga

When you've mastered these breathing techniques, take a hike or go for a swim. Both of these low-impact activities are ideal for people with HBV. Other low-impact ideas: yoga, dancing, biking, canoeing, gardening, chopping wood, mowing the lawn, walking in the mall, and last but certainly not least, sex.

Can I do more strenuous exercises?

Many people who I've interviewed have been told by their doctors to avoid exercise altogether. Ask your doctor to help set up exercise guidelines with you. If he isn't interested in discussing exercise or won't go into detail, ask him for a referral to a physical therapist for an hour consultation. If that doesn't work, call a trainer who has experience working with people with chronic conditions and make the investment.

In addition, the majority of my interviewees who are quite athletic say that they feel fine as long as they don't do too much exercise that involves cardio, or exercise that involves keeping your heart rate elevated for an extended period. I find that if I use the treadmill I can do up to 45 minutes at a brisk walk or slow jog, but I can't run for more that 10 minutes without feeling quite fatigued the next morning. This seems to be quite typical for many people with fibrosis, but you may find that you, like our skater Karin, have a high tolerance to strenuous exercise.

Of course, we all have different situations depending on our level of scarring, viral load, and liver enzymes. After discussing exercise with your health care professional, you will probably be better equipped to determine your own limits. The key, once again, is to start very slowly and gauge your own energy level and day-after consequences. After a few weeks or months you will almost certainly know what your body can handle.

The American Council on Exercise (ACE) is a nonprofit organization committed to promoting active, healthy lifestyles and their positive effects on the mind, body, and spirit. Their website has a health club search engine and excellent articles about exercise for those with chronic disease. Just click the "Fit Facts" button on the ACE website: http://www.acefitness.org/.

Getting into shape will help you to detoxify. And detoxifying will help you think more clearly and get a better night's sleep. Your liver will love it.

IN A SENTENCE:

> *Exercise is treatment.*

learning

Alternative Treatment

OVER 40 percent of Americans now use some form of complementary and alternative medicine, often called CAM for short. Believe it or not, there are now more patient visits each year to alternative practitioners than to conventional doctors, and even hospitals are now incorporating alternative practices into their medical system. Roughly 10 percent of all community hospitals in the United States now offer alternative treatments, and Americans now spend $30 billion annually on "unconventional" therapies.

In 1992 Congress created the National Center for Complementary and Alternative Medicine, a branch of the National Institutes of Health. Essentially, the NCCAM studies what works and what doesn't.

Herbs and stuff

Most conventional doctors aren't very well trained in nutrition, and even fewer have training in herbal supplements and alternative therapies. Nutritionists and dieticians are not always familiar with liver disease, so HBV patients often feel like they're left to fend for themselves. Well-known author Dr.

Andrew Weil suggests the following rule in his book *Spontaneous Healing* when deciding between conventional and alternative therapies: "Do not seek help from a conventional doctor for a condition that conventional medicine cannot treat, and do not rely on an alternative provider for a condition that conventional medicine can manage well."

That's good advice, but it's nonetheless hard to know whom to trust when it comes to herbs. Although interest is growing worldwide, we are still a few years away from sufficient studies of the efficacy of herbs for the liver. With the exception of milk thistle, which has been studied and used for decades, most claims that support the use of herbs are anecdotal, citing individual testimony rather than actual scientific trials. Also, herbs aren't regulated like pharmaceuticals, so the potency and efficacy of their active ingredients can vary widely from brand to brand.

If you would like more published information about herbal therapies, you can call the National Center for Complementary and Alternative Medicine (NCCAM) (301) 496-4000 or request faxes on demand directly and automatically at (888) 644-6226. The center's site is full of information and resources, and can be found at http://nccam/nih/gov.

Start slowly if you want to try using herbs

If you are interested in trying herbs, it's a good idea to ease into them very slowly. Check with your doctor before taking any supplements. Here are a few more suggestions:

- Don't use liver formulas which combine multiple herbs
- Don't try to prescribe Chinese medicine on your own
- Do a search and read about side effects and dosages
- Don't take herbal diet pills that promise swift weight loss
- Buy a reputable brand from a reputable store
- Avoid combining herbs with homeopathy, as they have contrasting philosophies (herbs fight symptoms, while homeopathy actually encourages the disease process)

Many people use milk thistle

The seeds of the milk thistle plant have been used for many years to protect the liver from toxins. Milk thistle contains compounds called syllimarin and sylibin that function as antioxidants and protect liver cells.

The recommended intake of milk thistle is 200–400mg daily. As mentioned above, make sure that you're taking pure milk thistle and not a blend of other herbs. Look for a respected brand.

Some take milk thistle every day as a supplement to traditional Western treatment (e.g., Lamivudine, Interferon). Milk thistle isn't exactly a medicine, but it is purported to help protect liver cells from damage induced by toxins. It has been used for many years in Europe, where some doctors even prescribe it. It is growing in popularity in the United States. Some hepatologists even recommend its use.

I tried taking milk thistle capsules before starting Lamivudine treatment, and my experience was positive, as I seroconverted during a period when I decided to try Dr. Andrew Weil's suggestions for hepatitis: milk thistle, schizandra (the fruit of *Schizandra chinensis*), low-fat mostly vegetarian diet and saunas. Of course we'll never know if this had anything to do with my seroconversion, but it did happen during the three-month period I followed his suggestions.

You can find the seeds in health food stores, and they can be toasted and eaten like pumpkin seeds. I've heard that the young leaves (with the spines removed) are edible, but I'll admit I haven't had the courage to try them.

Recent studies, however, show that milk thistle can slow down how quickly enzymes operate in the liver. For example, they may impede our ability to turn food into energy, or may intensify the side effects of traditional drugs. Too much milk thistle combined with Lamivudine could potentially raise the level of the drug in your system and be harmful. Other medications whose levels may increase due to milk thistle are:

Heart drugs: Tambocor, Rythmol
Antibiotics: Erythromycin, rifampin
Antiseizure drug: Carbamazepine
Antidepressants: Zyban/Wellbutrin, Paxil, Zoloft, Luvox, St. John's Wort, etc.
Other: Antifungals, antipsychotics, sedatives, and lipid-lowering drugs.

Check with your doctor before deciding to make milk thistle part of your daily regimen, and make sure you refresh his memory about other medications you're currently taking.

Other herbs are available, but none of them have been tested extensively

Dandelion. Chinese, Ayurvedic, Western herbalists, and traditional medical practitioners have all used dandelion for hepatitis over the centuries. The entire plant has been used either fresh, dried, cooked, or in a powder form. Some of us have even grown up eating the greens in our salads in springtime, though if you use weed killer or chemical fertilizers on your lawn, you will want to avoid putting homegrown dandelion on your table.

Dandelions have more vitamin A than raw carrots or spinach, so you won't want to go hog-wild on them. But therapeutically speaking they are slow acting and have anti-inflammatory and hepatotonic functions. Given that they are also a diuretic, you won't want to consume too much tea or greens before bedtime. In addition to eating the leaves, you can use the well-scrubbed root in your juicer as you would a carrot. Dandelion is available in capsules and teas as well.

Phyllanthus amarus is a flowering herb from India, where Ayurvedic practitioners have used it for many years to treat liver problems. The Chinese and Westerners have also conducted studies on it. Scientists have discovered compounds in the herb that fight HBV. It has been successfully tested in controlled studies, and in three of these trials it helped clear HBsAg in 60 percent of the participants. However, not all of these studies have proven its efficacy. An interesting note: the fruit of phyllanthus has 20 times more vitamin C than orange juice.

You will see phyllanthus on the shelves of your local health food store either alone or mixed with other herbs such as pirorhiza kurroa. Although at the present there are no known drug interactions with phyllanthus, you should be very careful about multiple herb combinations that may have interactions. It is used in the form of tea or in capsules.

Ginger has been used for thousands of years by the Chinese as a treatment for nausea. Those who are taking Interferon have found it to relieve chemotherapy-induced nausea. It is readily available and is also usually taken in the form of a tea. You can also use fresh ginger root in your cooking or steep fresh ginger shavings in hot water to make your own infusion.

Ginseng (Panax ginseng) has been used mostly to fight HBV-related fatigue and brain fog, but it is also a known immunomodulator, blood pressure and sugar regulator as well as sexual stimulant. It is one of the best-known herbs and has been used in China for thousands of years. Ginseng's action against HBV has been tested in vitro and in vivo with positive results. Great care should be used if taking ginseng, as there may be side effects such as high blood pressure, headaches, and nervous anxiety.

Licorice root (Glycyrrhiza glabra) is said to have both antiviral and anti-inflammatory properties, as well as immunomodulating activity. It has been thoroughly tested in human trials, some of which showed antiviral activity against HBV.

Licorice, unlike milk thistle, shouldn't be used for long periods, as it may cause high blood pressure, water retention, low potassium levels, or a disturbance in electrolyte balance. Herbalists urge caution against long-term treatment with it, and pregnant women or those with hypertension should not take it. Licorice has been used in Japan for many years, and studies there showed that it may help improve the condition of your liver and assist liver function. Licorice is usually taken in the form of a tea, but can also be found in capsules or powders.

Schizandra (Schizandra chinensis) is a vine and is native to China, where its sour red berries are cultivated and dried for use in decoctions and tinctures. In clinical trials it has helped to lower ALT in an average of 90 percent of those who took it, and it also helps increase glutathione production and minimize fatigue. Schizandra is quite safe to take and you can take it as you would milk thistle, in capsules or tablets, or you can buy dried berries from an herbalist or health food store and make your own herbal tea. Since Schizandra assists your immune system and has antioxidant liver protecting functions, herbalists also use it for night sweats, chronic coughing, and HIV.

Websites can help you find good brands and eliminate false claims

www.ConsumerLab.com is an independent lab that tests the quality of supplements. www.Quackwatch.com unmasks false claims. You can find more information from the American Botanical Council's website (http://www.herbalgram.org). The American Council on Science and Health runs an excellent site (http://www.acsh.org), as does The National Council Against Health Fraud (http://www.ncahf.org/). See the resources section at the end of this book for recommended reading on herbs.

You must avoid some herbs altogether

The following herbs are hepatotoxic:

○ Chaparral
○ Comfrey (bush tea)
○ Germander
○ Echinacea
○ Ephedrine
○ Jin bu huan
○ Kava
○ Nutmeg
○ Pennyroyal oil
○ Ma Huang
○ Mistletoe
○ Tansy ragwort
○ Sassafras
○ Senna
○ Skullcap
○ Valerian
○ Yerba tea

Homeopathy

A German physician named Samuel Hahnemann developed a treatment strategy called Homeopathy in the 1800s with the simple idea that "like cures like," and that highly diluted quantities of these substances—herbs, chemicals, minerals, and animal products—could reverse the symptoms of disease that they, in turn, induce. This may seem like Western science turned on its head, but homeopathy has had loyal followers for over 200 years. Although homeopathy does involve the use of herbs, it is quite different than herbal medicine since these diluted substances contain nearly undetectable amounts (as little as 1 part in a trillion) of active ingredients.

Homeopathy is a **holistic** field of medicine, meaning that it involves not just biology but personality and lifestyle. Hahnemann identified principal human personality types, each with its own propensity for certain diseases and discomforts. Homeopaths, like reiki therapists, sometimes refer to their remedies as "energy imprints" that potentiate the body's "vital forces." No one denies that part of its healing power comes from this almost poetic and noninvasive nature, and we all know the power of believing when it comes to healing.

Clinical studies have shown that homeopathic remedies have more of an effect than placebos (sugar pills) and, since homeopathic remedies are so diluted, they are safe to mix and match or combine with traditional medicines. In fact, you can find them (often in lipstick-size containers) at your local health food store or pharmacy next to herbal remedies. Their labels do, however, specify ingredients, dosage, degree of dilution, and a description of their intended use. Some purists avoid this tendency, but none would suggest treating serious diseases with homeopathy and nothing else.

Avoid self-diagnosis. If you do find a reputable homeopath, you may get a prescription for some of these more common remedies for hepatitis:

phosphorous
hepar sulph
lycopodium
podophyllum
medorrhinum
chelidonium
lachesis
nux vomica

Although I no longer use homeopathic medicine, I did before my HBV diagnosis. I turned to homeopathy to help with what I believed was simply chronic fatigue. My personal experience with homeopathy over eight years in Europe was positive.

Reiki: Healing hands and positive energy

Although it has its origin in India, reiki is a Japanese word meaning "universal life force energy," and is used now to describe a hands-on healing therapy. Reiki employs the use of stimulating hands that are positioned over the body to promote healing. The art of reiki is passed from mentor to apprentice via mystic initiations called attunements or empowerments that engage the universal life force energy. It works by replacing your negative energy with the positive "vibratory frequencies."

Reiki is becoming more popular in the United States, and hepatitis may be one of the more ideal diseases for this approach. Simply by positioning hands above your liver, a reiki therapist draws energy inside your liver and calms your mind and spirit. Since a successful reiki session will release tension in your body, it is thought that it can help eliminate toxins and waste products from your body. Given that positive energy is its main driving force, reiki may not work for you if you consciously or unconsciously believe that it cannot work for you, or if you feel guilty or believe that you deserve your illness.

Reiki can be a good accompaniment to conventional treatment, along with diet, exercise and meditation. You can even try self-treatment by cupping both your hands over your liver as you lie on your bed in a warm, low-lit room, sending positive energy and warmth to your liver. You can also ask your partner to join you in weekly sessions. Trained professionals believe that you really need experience to gain the full effect, but who knows—you might just have a knack for harnessing the universal life force energy.

Chinese Medicine

Like homeopathy, Chinese medicine is holistic, but it differs from it in that over the centuries it has evolved into a study of the body's harmony, or lack thereof. This harmony or equilibrium is governed by specific groups of interconnected organs and what the Chinese call essential substances that give us energy and emotions. In fact, Chinese medicine does not distinguish between the body and the spirit of a human being. Organs are divided into yin (interior) and yang (exterior) groups. The liver, in case you're wondering, is in the yin category.

If you decide to use CM (Chinese Medicine), you have to change your Western expectations and attitudes. For example, you shouldn't expect to just pop a pill or brew a pot of tea and be fixed. Your CM practitioner may help you radically change your ideas about managing chronic illness. You may be asked to do **acupuncture**, herbal therapy, Qi Gong exercise, and meditation.

Since the practice is quite involved and deserves much more in-depth illustration than can be provided in the scope of this book, I hope you will search out the following excellent resources:

Doc Misha's Chicken Soup Chinese Medicine site
Misha Cohen, O.M.D., L.Ac
E-mail: chinmedsf@aol.com
http://www.docmisha.com

Acupuncture.com
www.acupuncture.com

American Association of Oriental Medicine (AAOM)
433 Front Street
Catasauqua, PA 18032-2506
(610) 266-1433
www.aaom.org (in-depth referral database)

Acupuncture and Oriental Medicine Alliance
14637 Starr Road S.E.
Olalla, WA 98539
(253) 851-6896
http://www.acupuncturealliance.org/

IN A SENTENCE:

> *There are other, more holistic or natural strategies for treating HBV,
> however they have not been thoroughly tested in controlled studies;
> if you want to try CAM you should find a professional licensed
> alternative practitioner.*

FIRST-MONTH MILESTONE

By the end of your first month, you're taking steps to proactively improve your quality of life due to your better understanding of how to:

○ CHOOSE THE RIGHT FOODS FOR YOUR LIVER.

○ DEAL WITH EMOTIONAL ISSUES TIED WITH LIVING WITH A CHRONIC DISEASE.

○ MAKE A GOOD DECISION ABOUT TREATMENT OPTIONS.

○ AVOID TOXINS THAT CAN HARM YOUR LIVER.

Diet:
Phase Out

YOU'D THINK that with 400 million HBV people in the world someone could come up with a reliable diet regimen for us. However, no one seems to know exactly what people with liver disease should eat. The stock phrases "discuss your diet with your doctor" or "eat a well-balanced meal with fresh fruits and vegetables" are vague almost to the point of being dismissive, and we just don't get a clear idea of what we really should and shouldn't be putting in our mouths. It's also hard to avoid the onslaught of saturated fats, sodium, and sugar that we're offered by franchises and convenience stores. My dream for all of us is that someone will soon open a nationwide chain called The Happy Hepper where you can get whole grain foods, an organic salad bar, and sugar-free desserts. And not a globule of hydrogenated oil in sight.

Our own idea of what constitutes "well-balanced" is also, at times, unreliable, and it varies widely from person to person. For one, it may mean no processed or genetically altered foods and only organically grown produce, while for another it means having a diet Coke and a Whopper-hold-the-mayo.

To be fair, the liver has different nutritional requirements for each phase of HBV. Many of us also have to juggle other ailments like diabetes or heart disease, each with its own special considerations. Although it is true that we're all different and that our diet also depends on what kind of condition our liver is in, it is worthwhile to have a more specific idea for those without damage, those with fibrosis, and those with cirrhosis. The bottom line here is that the critical regimen for those who have fibrosis and cirrhosis laid out in this chapter can be adopted as a purely preventative measure for those who are asymptomatic or in the early stages of HBV.

After gaining a basic understanding of the basic fundamentals of nutrition, you will then have to gauge both what tastes good and what makes you feel good. Talk to other people with HBV and find out what works for them. If you do ask for a referral to see a nutritionist, try and find one who has experience with liver disease.

We covered basics of nutrition and basic components in Week 2. Now let's cover strategies for eating right so we can take care of our livers.

Gradually phase out unhealthy food

Taking that first step towards altering your diet is hard. Sometimes we just have to take baby steps. I've come to call the initial entry into the world of HBV dining the phase-out period. It's the phase in which you realize that you need to thoroughly alter your eating habits and find the courage and energy to break bad habits.

Phasing out is a kind of 12-step program that helps you progressively alter your diet step by step. Having to do this when you're single is hard enough, but having to avoid foods when you have a healthy herd to cook for is very hard. If you have a strong will and can change at the drop of a spoon, you're lucky. This program is made for those of us who have serious inbred cravings for beef jerky and red licorice. The basic idea of the phase-out diet is to take one component of your diet at a time and make it undergo a progressive division by halves. This gradual decrease must then be counterbalanced by healthful substitutes. Over the next few months you will be able to choose which of these dietary components you want to work on. You may find it helpful to work on one at a time if your eating habits are entrenched. Otherwise double up and tackle two or more at a time if you can.

The basic components you will need to work on are: alcohol, trans/saturated fats, red meat, nicotine, sugar, sugar substitutes, salt, preservatives and food coloring, and unfiltered tap water. It may sound ludicrous, but those of us who have worked hard to lessen our suffering from fatigue and brain fog say it's the only way. You will too once you've taken the first few steps. Denny Norton agrees: "I've gotten to where I don't feel well eating much fat at all. I get nausea, headaches, and fatigue within 10 minutes of eating anything high in fat. I'm now feeling better, since I have gotten stricter with staying low fat. I hate it, but it has helped me a lot."

This phase-out period will also help your taste buds gradually adjust. If you stay on target with the progressive removal of fats, sugars, and chemicals from your diet, you will notice that your taste buds adjust to the new, healthful choices you're making. It will become difficult to return to your old ways once you're gained some momentum.

Accordingly, your first phase out priority must absolutely be alcohol.

Quickly eliminate alcohol consumption

Alcohol is actually thought to aid replication of HBV, in addition to being toxic and causing extra work for the liver. If you are now accustomed to enjoying a glass of wine or two with dinner every night, here is a sample schedule for phasing out alcohol that may seem reasonable to you.

This week:	1 glass with dinner 2 times per week
Next week:	½ glass with dinner 2 times per week
Next month:	½ glass per month
Ongoing:	Enough to wet your lips for a toast at major holidays and special events

This is only a suggestion if you feel stressed about facing this challenge. Otherwise it would be far more preferable to stop today. Many people say that they feel so much better after a few months that they no longer desire alcohol.

If you think that you might not be able to stop on your own, skip ahead to Month 9 for more information.

Minimize your intake of saturated fats and hydrogenated oil/trans fats

You see this ingredient on all kinds of products, but what exactly is it? In the **hydrogenation** process, oil is literally sprayed through hydrogen, altering the molecular structure by adding hydrogen atoms. It turns oil into a semisolid substance that is so very essential to modern foods that strive for perfect texture. In fact, hydrogenation prevents oil from becoming rancid for centuries. Well maybe not centuries, but regardless, for the HBV diet it's a disaster. Studies show that it stays in our systems longer than regular fat, and seems to promote arterial plaque. It may deplete the supply of vitamin E in our bodies and can raise the levels of LDL cholesterol levels in our blood. The FDA has toyed with the idea of labeling guidelines for hydrogenated oils and trans fats, so that they can't be hidden in the foods you eat. The word is slowly getting out.

Next time you go to the supermarket, have a closer look at labels. Good luck finding foods made without hydrogenated or partially hydrogenated oil! Nearly every cookie, bread, cracker, cereal, stuffing, creamer, and snack has it. Once, I searched high and low for some kind of snack that I could eat while at the computer. I brought home a bag of trail mix, thinking it was a healthy choice. Then I looked at the ingredients. Hydrogenated oil had been sprayed onto the raisins and nuts, along with blue and red food coloring. I could have cried.

Years ago someone posted an article from a health journal about hydrogenated oil on the fridge at my office. It listed a series of symptoms that may possibly be induced by eating too much hydrogenated oil: aches, headaches, joint aches, fuzzy thinking. Just about the same symptoms that someone with HBV suffers. The article suggested eliminating hydrogenated oils from your diet for one month to see if there was a noticeable decrease in symptoms. I did it for a month and have continued with the diet ever since. That was seven years ago. Having lived abroad for ten years, I used to return to the States every summer for a few weeks to visit family. I could never understand why I would always get headaches and fuzzy thoughts within days of returning. And when I'd return to Italy these symptoms would disappear. Now I'm convinced that the trans fats were the culprits. At that time there weren't nearly as many foods being made with hydrogenated oils in Italy. After exercise, removing hydrogenated oil from my diet was perhaps the single most significant thing I did to lessen fatigue and brain fog.

Try to choose oils that are produced organically. Look for the words "cold pressed" or "expeller pressed" on the label as these oils are obtained through a natural process. Some oils on the supermarket shelf are produced with the help of solvents. Avoid these—we don't need any more toxins in our bodies than we already have. Keep the lid tightly sealed on the oil and replace oils that have been in open dispensers too long, as they can go bad over time.

Cut down on full-fat dairy products

Since 1970 Americans have doubled their intake of cheese. We now eat 27 pounds per person per year on average. That's over half a pound per week. Those with HBV should be eating far less—just a few ounces of full-fat cheese per week.

Switch to skim or nonfat milk. Although you may think that 2 percent milk means that the milk only has 2 percent fat, it means that by weight it is only 2 percent. Try cooking with soy or rice milk in recipes that call for a lot of milk. There are dozens of low fat or nonfat cheese or veggie cheeses. If you can't avoid full-fat cheese, eat small amounts infrequently. A few slices of processed cheese can have as much as eight grams of fat. It's probably better to avoid blue cheese and other full-fat cheeses.

Most of our annual cheese consumption is from the mozzarella on pizza, and though a pizza party is infinitely tempting, the saturated fat content weighs heavily on your liver. Some of us with fibrosis and cirrhosis joke about wearing our pizza an hour after eating it, as the fat seems to go straight to the pores of the skin on our faces. To minimize this effect, avoid extra-cheese pizzas, deep-dish cheese pizzas, and those with cheese-stuffed crusts. Look for reduced fat or reduced sodium pizzas, or make your own. Of course pizza without cheese is not pizza, so if you can't avoid it, eat it once a month and mop up some of the surface oil with a paper towel after it has cooled a few minutes.

Do not eat raw or undercooked fish or shellfish

Although seafood is easy to digest, generally low in fat and a healthy alternative to red meat, eating raw or even undercooked shellfish can be deadly when you have liver disease. Bacteria called vibrios and something called the Norwalk virus can multiply in fish, even after refrigeration. Vibrios can be killed only when the seafood is thoroughly cooked. For this reason, you must not eat any of the following uncooked: fin fish, oysters, scallops, shellfish, clams, mussels, and mollusks. Sushi and sashimi are relatively safe for people without liver disease because the fish used to make them have been frozen at subzero temperatures, which kills any parasites. However, this low temperature does not kill bacteria, leaving people with hepatitis B particularly vulnerable. Thorough cooking, however, will kill both parasites and bacteria.

Minimize your intake of red meat and cured meats

It's a good idea to avoid too much bacon, sausage, luncheon meats, or other cured meats. Avoid raw meat as well. Not only do they contain nitrates and copious amounts of sodium, but also they have saturated fat and are hard to digest. They are the second leading source of fats and the fourth leading source of saturated fat in American diets. Substitute vegetarian versions, or switch to turkey, chicken, or fish whenever possible. Make it a special end-of-the-month treat to go have your customary Sunday brunch and limit intake of red meat to once or twice a month. Trim it well, eat small portions, and don't eat it too late in the evening. Liver and onions is great on a cold January night, but the dish has too much iron for your own liver to handle.

Eliminate as much sugar as you can

Your liver tries its best to regulate sugar levels in your blood, especially between meals. But if you have fibrosis or cirrhosis and drink or eat too much sugar on an empty stomach you may get a sugar high and then crash about twenty minutes later. Sometimes severe liver disease can cause hypo-glycemia—low blood sugar—in which very low blood glucose levels bring about certain symptoms like sweating, shaking, light-headedness, and hunger.

If this sounds like you, you may want to avoid consuming candy, sugary drinks, and rich desserts. If you can't do without it, try eating them only after meals, so that the sugar will enter your bloodstream more gradually. But remember, when your blood sugar is high your liver converts excess sugar into stored glycogen or even fat.

Bottom line: Consuming large quantities of sugar when you have liver disease is like driving on an icy road—you may spin out of control and crash.

Avoid dietary mind games

It's easy to fall prey to mind games regarding food and alcohol when you have HBV. For example, if we feel we're being good about not drinking, we may decide we can be bad with nicotine or fatty foods. It's human to want to reward ourselves for hard work or accomplishment. Unfortunately, most of our rewards involve alcohol and saturated fat consumption. To avoid this trap, get into the habit of rewarding yourself with a day off work, a nap, music, a new book, or a walk in the woods.

Be realistic about phasing out

If and when these changes seem overwhelming to you and/or your family, break them down and separate them in your mind. Make a list if you think it will help. Decide which of the items on your list need immediate attention or seem more within your immediate reach. Invite your partner to see the list and discuss what things can be mutually beneficial to both of you and which your partner or family can't do without.

Chances are good that by the end of the phase-out you will feel comfortable with and proud of your progress, and you may even be encouraged to move on to further refinements such as cutting down on salt, preservatives, or caffeine. As you gain momentum, you will begin to understand that in order to keep your liver happy your diet requires the kinds of dietary exchanges that diabetics must follow. If you have a heavy meal in a restaurant one night, you may want to keep it light and simple the next, all the while drinking plenty of water or herbal tea.

Think twice about sugar substitutes

It seems that every few years we read stories about how unhealthy artificial sweeteners are. Billions of diet drinks have been consumed over the past 25 years since these additives made their way into our foods and, with the exception of saccharin (since removed from the U.S. government's list of known carcinogens), no safety issues have emerged from their use. Of course, this doesn't mean that there aren't any safety issues, or that we won't discover down the road that it can lead to diseases such as multiple sclerosis, Lou Gehrig's disease, or other disorders. A flood of conjecture about possible side effects has popped up on websites and in consumers' psyches.

The bottom line right now is that (1) there *are* chemicals involved, and (2) we don't know enough to feel really comfortable about ingesting these substances, since it could take decades to trace and document harm. Nutrasweet®, for example, is metabolized into formaldehyde in your body, though in tiny amounts (i.e., maybe you just embalm a cell or two with every drink).

Sweeteners make me feel edgy and uncomfortable. After having avoided them for the past twenty years, I decided this year to let down my guard and see what I was missing. I had to stop after a few weeks. I had mild headaches and felt stiffness in my joints. When I stopped, they disappeared. If you experience similar symptoms and have any suspicions that artificial sweeteners might be the cause, try stopping for a few weeks. You can always go back if you don't notice a difference.

Bottom line: No one knows for sure. But a damaged liver can't remove these chemicals as quickly or as effectively as a healthy liver.

Avoid added salt

Salt is present in fruits, vegetables, nuts, and seeds, sources which supply us with all the salt our bodies really need. Natural sodium sources offer a more complex form that is absorbed more slowly than refined table salt.

When we send too much sodium into our bloodstream, the body stores it between cells until our kidneys are able to filter it. The cells aren't too happy about the extra salt, so they release water into the fluid in an attempt to dilute it. However, when these cells expel water, they lose elasticity and shrivel, resulting in a loss of potassium.

We hear a lot about low-sodium diets. Typically these diets recommend no more than 2–3 grams (2000–3000 milligrams) of sodium per day. Unfortunately, many Americans consume more than 10,000 mg of salt daily. Just one pickle has over 1,000 mg, and a can of soup can have 500 mg or more. Check labels carefully, and if you see the word "healthy" on a label it means that the food contains less than 480 milligrams of sodium per serving. Soda, which is actually sodium bicarbonate (baking soda) and sodium (symbol Na) refers to sodium compounds. Many water-softening systems use sodium as the softening agent. If you have a water softener and drink tap water, you may want to bypass the water faucet in the kitchen.

You'll need a few weeks to adjust to less salt, but your taste bud receptors do eventually adjust. Those of us with leg edema, ascites, or high blood pressure should definitely reduce sodium intake.

A recent study by Johns Hopkins University, however, shows that salt actually reduces the symptoms of fatigue. A few people with HBV who I've interviewed have expressed an actual craving for salt. This is probably because after consuming salt their blood pressure goes up and they feel temporarily more alert and awake.

Bottom line: You get enough salt from foods, and too much can make you dehydrated and affect your blood pressure.

What's up with peanuts and peanut butter?

There is conflicting information about whether peanuts are safe to eat when you have hepatitis, since they may contain by-products of mold that can grow on nuts and grains. These by-products are called **aflatoxins**, and improper storage conditions are usually to blame. Most industrialized nations regulate aflatoxin levels in food, but aflatoxin can also be passed to humans via milk and meat. In the United States, peanuts are carefully checked for aflatoxin contamination during the manufacturing process.

For this reason, it is wise to steer clear of stale, discolored, or moldy nuts of any kind. Also, while travelling, try to avoid nuts or even rice in countries where food regulations may not be carried out so stringently. Furthermore, don't leave peanut butter or other grains uncovered for long periods of time. Store them in a cool dry place to avoid mold, and throw them away if you can't remember when you purchased them.

Most mainstream peanut butter brands contain a small amount of partially hydrogenated oil, which keeps the oil from separating from the peanut butter and gives the peanut butter a creamier texture. Shelf life is also extended. Although you may not find it in your mainstream grocery store, try to buy natural peanut butters. The oil may rise to the top and it may not last on the shelf for ten years, but your heart and liver will thank you for the extra effort.

Bottom line: You can still eat peanuts if you're not allergic to them. Just make sure the peanuts are fresh and your peanut butter doesn't contain hydrogenated oil.

Your cooking methods are important

Cooking can cut down the amount of vitamins found naturally in foods. For this reason it's a good idea to use small amounts of water and avoid overcooking. Use nonfat cooking spray or an olive oil sprayer, or use nonstick pans. Eating a few raw meals per week is a good way to help avoid fat.

Iron skillets: If your ferritin (iron) levels are in the normal range, you probably needn't worry about cooking in your old iron skillet. If your iron is high or you want to stay on the safe side, you may want to find a different pan. Then again, you may just want to hide your frying pan altogether.

Microwave ovens: If you must use your microwave, only use glass or ceramic containers as microwaves can drive foreign molecules into the food in plastic containers. Transfer frozen food into glass or ceramic too. Do not overcook! Microwaves retain nearly as much water and vitamins in the food as standard cooking methods, but overcooking will zap too many of the vitamins. Some people find that getting rid of the microwave altogether helps improve their diet. To find out if this in true in your case, write down a list of all the foods that you regularly heat in the microwave. Chances are good that most of them will be high in fat and sodium.

Steaming is a very liver-friendly way to cook. If you grill meat, be sure to remove the skin and extra fat, and cover the meat with barbeque sauce or marinade, as it will cut down on the amount of toxins that enter the meat on the grill.

Cirrhosis demands that you be even more careful

As if all this phasing out stuff wasn't enough, if you have cirrhosis you need to be even more careful. You may even experience a loss of appetite and increased fatigue with more advanced liver damage. Here a few common considerations:

Protein: Cirrhosis has a love/hate relationship with protein: too little, and it could affect body functions, your energy level, and it could even result in a loss of muscle. Too much protein, however, can lead to encephalopathy, or brain swelling. Talk to your doctor about finding a realistic balance, or ask to see a dietician that has experience with cirrhosis. It's usually a good idea to limit protein to small portions consumed in more frequent yet smaller meals. You can get plenty of protein even if you don't eat any meat, but you should do some research to find the best alternative sources. Limit or eliminate full-fat dairy products. And don't overdo it with soy products—they contain phyto-estrogens that can modulate your hormone production.

Vitamins and minerals: Many of those with cirrhosis take vitamin supplements, as long as they aren't huge doses. Cirrhosis can cause deficiencies, particularly in calcium, zinc, and magnesium.

Sugar: When cirrhosis is present, your liver has an even harder time juggling your glucose levels. This can cause either high blood sugar (hyperglycemia) or low blood sugar (hypoglycemia). For this reason you'll want to avoid heavy doses of simple sugars like candy, desserts, and soft drinks. Some people find that eating small doses of simple sugars after a meal avoids the sugar rush followed by a crash and burn, or sudden drop in energy.

Salt: Too much salt will increase your chance of developing ascites and bloating. Your doctor will limit sodium intake to no more than 2000 mg per day. Avoiding salt will very likely be one of your key challenges, as most packaged foods and fast foods have exceedingly high sodium levels. Be aware that even breakfast cereals and desserts can have added sodium. If you are still retaining fluid in your abdomen or ankles, your doctor may ask you to take a diuretic like Lasix or Aldactone. If you are taking diuretics, you may also need to take potassium supplements as diuretics flush it out of your body.

Fat: Be even more careful to avoid as many saturated and trans fats as possible, and avoid full-fat dairy products.

IN A SENTENCE:

> *Gradually phasing out certain foods while counterbalancing them with healthful substitutes will help your immune systems and liver function in an optimal way whether you have liver scarring or not.*

learning

The HBV Vaccine

*The HBV vaccine
is the first anticancer treatment*

AS DISCUSSED in Day 2, the blood test for HBV was discovered by Dr. Baruch Blumberg in 1965. Just four years later, Blumberg invented the HBV vaccine along with Irving Millman. This early vaccine was called inactivated hepatitis B vaccine because it used a heat-treated form of the antigen. This vaccine was found not to be infectious but immunogenic, meaning it triggered a response from the immune system. Development of the HBV vaccine got a boost in 1973 when HBV was successfully transmitted in experiments involving chimpanzees, and this led to the development of a generation of plasma-derived vaccines. These vaccines were developed by painstakingly gathering antibodies from the blood of those who had already recovered from hepatitis B. A second generation of genetically engineered or recombinant DNA vaccines is now used around the world, so that there is no longer a risk of transmitting other human infections via the serum-based vaccine.

The normal schedule for HBV vaccination is three shots over six months. A great deal of protection is offered by the first shot (over 50 percent of those who get the first shot develop immunity), but complete protection usually occurs only after the final injection. However, the older you are when you get the vaccine, the greater your chances are of not developing immunity. Those who receive their first HBV vaccine after age 40 or over may want to have their doctor check to make sure they've developed antibodies after the full series. The effect of the HBV vaccine also appears to decrease in obese people and in those who are on **hemodialysis**.

The HBV vaccine has the honor of being the first official anticancer vaccine.

Who needs to get it?

The American College of International Physicians (ACIP) recommends universal vaccination of newborns, children, and adolescents. Others at high risk are recipients of blood products like people with an inherited form of anemia called thallasemia, those undergoing hemodialysis, IV drug users, those who work with young children, family contacts and sex partners of those with HBV infection, health workers and those who work in laboratories, and, of course, nurses and doctors. Those with multiple sex partners should also get the vaccine and cross at least one transmissible disease off their list, though of course it goes without saying that we can get HBV from even just one sex partner. Persons who plan to travel to areas that have high HBV rates should be vaccinated, as well as people who will be performing medical procedures in areas where HBV infection is common, who are at very high risk.

For obvious reasons those with chronic HBV tend to be quite vocal about the need for everyone to get the shots. We do our best to get the word out.

Extensive trials of these recombinant vaccines have proven safe, effective, and free of side effects (with the exception of soreness at the injection site). If you live in the United States, the vaccine will cost you or your insurance company about $150. If you live abroad where both government and pharmaceutical companies subsidize the vaccine, you may pay as little as $5.

Those who have had a full vaccination series are protected against HBV infection; however, your close family or partner may need to check their antibody levels to ensure that they have protective levels (>10 units/ml). Unless their levels fall below this level, they will not need to receive a booster dose of the vaccine.

Mistakes are sometimes made in the administration of vaccines

Check to make sure your partner and friends receive the complete series. My interviewees have told stories about incomplete shots or shots that were given on the wrong schedule. One of my friends even received an HBV vaccine on the first month and HAV shots in the months that followed. The error was discovered only by accident. Take responsibility for making sure all the shots are given, that they are given at the proper time, and that the right vaccines are being used.

The HBV vaccine schedule for adults is as follows:

FIRST HBV SHOT	SECOND HBV SHOT	THIRD HBV SHOT
initial injection	1–2 months after first shot MUST BE AT LEAST 4 WEEKS AFTER FIRST SHOT	2–5 months after first shot MUST BE AT LEAST 4 MONTHS AFTER SECOND SHOT

By contrast, the hepatitis A vaccine consists of two injections 6 months apart.

The most common brands of HBV vaccine are **Engerix-B** (SmithKline) and Recombivax-HB (Merck). The original plasma-derived vaccine, named Heptavax, is no longer available in the United States.

Government intervention and private endowments make a difference

The HBV vaccine is now available all over the world. Outside the United States, pharmaceutical companies have pooled resources with local governments to make the vaccine available to a wide audience for less than $10. And the Bill and Melinda Gates Foundation has given hundreds of millions of dollars to make sure the vaccine reaches even the poorest nations. This is a generous and important donation that we don't hear enough about. It will save millions of livers and lives. Their website is full of useful information, including a concise and clearly written hepatitis B fact sheet. You can visit the site at www.childrensvaccine.org.

Your immune system has a built-in memory for antigens

It is commonly held belief that people who were vaccinated more than ten years ago should receive a booster shot of HBV vaccine. However, your body has a built-in memory for HBV, so it is thought that anyone who received the vaccine and is exposed to the virus will have developed enough antibodies to fight off the virus, even if their antibody levels (or **titres**) are quite low. This is called an anamnestic response. It is probably a good idea for your partner or family to have their titres checked, but you may want to discuss the need for booster shots with your doctor.

Some HBV negative people should check antibodies regularly

Booster shots of HBV vaccine are not usually necessary, given that protection is thought to last a lifetime, but people with HIV or kidney disease or those with impaired immune systems should have regular testing of their antibodies (some recommend annually) to make sure that the level does not drop below 10 IU/ml.

Unfortunately, not everyone develops antibodies after getting the vaccine. Five percent of newborns and young children do not develop a sufficient quantity of antibodies after receiving the full vaccine series. This could be due to genetics, infection, a compromised immune system due to the presence of HIV or other diseases. This is yet another reason why it is a good idea to check titres.

Some people are trying the vaccine as treatment

Vaccine therapy is what we call the use of the HBV vaccine as treatment. Recent animal studies have shown that administering the vaccine to those already infected with HBV can induce seroconversion and the development of the s antibody. This is great news, at least for the lucky 20 percent of those in the study. There is at least one documented success story of vaccine-induced human seroconversion in Europe.

This experimental treatment strategy isn't for everyone. Experts suggest that vaccine therapy may be an option only for those who have managed to sustain no or low viral load for at least a year. Vaccine therapy is thought to be safe, since thousands every year unknowingly receive the vaccine despite prior and ongoing HBV infection. Some hepatologists suggest a double dose administered on an accelerated schedule of first dose followed by booster shots at month 1 and 2.

Triple antigen vaccines (Hepacare, **Medeva**) have been shown to be more effective because they contain extra molecules against which an antibody will be produced and to which it will bind. These are called **epitopes**, and those for HBV are called S, *pre S1* and *pre S2* antigens. It is thought that more varieties of antigens in the vaccine will increase the chance that you will develop antibodies to lock into them. Unfortunately, although these vaccines are in clinical trials, they are not yet available in the United States.

Some people refuse to let their children get it

A woman in Arkansas refused to let her children be vaccinated, saying they are not at risk because they are not sexually active and don't do drugs, and getting the vaccine would give the impression that her children were promiscuous or drug abusers. A man in New Jersey refused to let his son get the vaccine because he thinks it's a ploy the pharmaceutical companies use to make more money. He says hepatitis is a "junkie's disease" and, as such, is unwarranted for young kids. It's hard to reason with ignorance, but someone should introduce them to the millions of kids who are infected with HBV at birth or early childhood and who also happen to share playgrounds with their children. Those who are concerned about the vaccine should contact the IAC, CDC, or Hepatitis B Foundation for more information and statistics. See Resources.

Some of the bad rap the HBV vaccine receives is due, in part, to bad press about one of its ingredients. Thimerosal—a preservative that was routinely added to a variety of vaccines—contains mercury and, although there is no proof that small doses of thimerosal caused any harm, it has, since 2000, been replaced by other preservatives.

Would you like hepatitis fries with that?

Studies are now being carried out to deliver the hepatitis B vaccine via genetically engineered produce like tomatoes, corn, and potatoes. Jokingly called pharming, this new procedure actually implants human genes into vegetables to grow antibodies that can be inexpensively extracted and turned into profit. One company is producing a contraceptive by splicing a genetic human defect into corn in order to make the plant generate a protein that kills sperm.

It is important to get the hepatitis A vaccine

If you have never had hepatitis A, you should get vaccinated. Co-infection with HBV and HAV can put your liver at serious risk. If you're not sure or can't remember if you had it as a child, your doctor can check you for HAV antibodies the next time you do your regular testing. Like HBV, if you've ever had it and cleared it, your body has developed antibodies to it and your immune system will kick in to fight it. Roughly half of Americans have been exposed to it at some time in their lives, and abroad those numbers skyrocket. We may feel that food handling and hygiene is so good in the United States that we needn't worry. However, it is exactly for this reason that we are unprotected, since many of us have never been previously exposed to the virus.

You can get complete protection from hepatitis A with just two injections administered six months apart. Not many primary physicians will ask if you've ever had the vaccine, so it is a good idea to request either a check of HAV antibodies or the vaccine itself. There is also a new combination HAV/HBV vaccine that you can recommend to your family and friends.

IN A SENTENCE:

> The first anticancer vaccine won the Nobel Prize for Dr. Baruch Blumberg, and is sometimes used as treatment in clinical trials; you must get the hepatitis A vaccine if you have HBV.

MONTH **3**

living

Sex,
Relationships,
and Esteem

*Safe sex is even more important
when you have HBV*

LATELY, THE CDC has come under fire for keeping quiet
about the true effectiveness (or lack thereof) of condoms. In
fact, organizations representing 25,000 physicians across the
United States outright accused the Centers for Disease Control
and Prevention of a cover-up. Twenty years have passed since
we first heard about HIV, and the message sent to the masses
over the years was that condoms would effectively protect us
from disease. We may have been given a false sense of security.
In retrospect, given increasing numbers of aggressive viruses
like HBV, HPV (human papillomavirus), chlamydia, syphilis,
trichomoniasis, and genital herpes—which can potentially be
transmitted *despite* condom use—this message seems, at best,
inadequate. Use a condom? Yes. But use your head too.

Those with HBV are at greater risk for contracting HIV

Unfortunately, people with HBV are more prone to contracting other viruses since our immune systems are already challenged. And HBV/HIV co-infection may make it tougher for you to get a new liver (should you need it), since co-infection may lessen the likelihood of successful transplantation and/or posttransplant treatment. In other words, practicing safe sex isn't just about not infecting others with HBV; it is also about protecting your chances of getting a liver if and when you should ever need it.

Some people think that because an HIV viral load is undetectable, there is no risk of HIV transmission. Unfortunately, this is not the case. Studies show that blood levels of HIV may not accurately predict the amount of HIV in semen, so it is possible to have an undetectable viral load in your blood and a detectable viral load in your semen. And it is possible to contract HIV through oral sex.

Don't combine drugs and sex

You can listen to all the rock and roll you want, but it probably won't surprise you to know that recreational drugs are the leading cause of unsafe sex. If you're high, the last thing you're thinking about is a condom. Sharing straws for snorting cocaine or sharing IV needles can pass HBV on to your fellow partiers, and drugs like Viagra make men very effective transmitters of HBV, especially when combined with speed or alcohol. In addition, combining Viagra with poppers (nitrates) causes blood vessels to dilate too much, possibly leading to strokes or heart attacks. In a recent study, men who take Viagra reported having twice as many partners as those who did not use the drug.

When you're high you're also more likely to share sex toys or other sexual accoutrements where traces of blood or bodily fluids can be found.

Kissing is safe, but avoid breaking world records

Kissing, as many of us know, is quite a pleasant way to pass a rainy afternoon. Or any afternoon for that matter. But sometimes when you have a contagious disease it's hard to find pleasure in it, particularly if you're concerned about infecting the person in such close and tantalizing proximity. Not only are we distracted by the thought of infecting others, but those with cirrhosis may also have chronic bad breath, gum disease, or **glossitis**.

Unfortunately, bleeding from the gums seems to be quite common among those with HBV. Flossing, use of an electric or water jet toothbrush, and more frequent visits to the dental hygienist will help minimize bleeding.

If your viral load is quite high, you may want to avoid deeply kissing someone who may not have had the vaccine or recovered from a prior HBV infection. Saliva can transmit HBV in active HBV infection, particularly when small amounts of blood are present. This fact has not been adequately communicated. Some reports claim that kissing does not transmit HBV, but don't place your bets on it. Doing your thorough brushing early in the morning is a good way to minimize risk if you have a hot date in the evening.

Kissing us can make some people nervous. Ray is a college student: "Growing up with hepatitis never caused any problems with anyone until my freshman year of college. I was dating a girl and she freaked when she saw a poster in the university health clinic saying you can catch hep B from kissing. That led to a good-bye which turned out to be for the best anyway."

If your partner has ever had and recovered from HBV or had the HBV vaccine, you can relax about your fears of infecting him or her.

Estrogen birth control and testosterone usage should be monitored

Consult with your specialist before using oral contraceptives or estrogens. The same caution should be used with methyltestosterone (testosterone), a male hormone.

I don't want you to see me like this

When you care about someone, you wish only good things for him or her. So it may seem logical to wish that your partner or child not witness what you imagine will be the slow and unpleasant degradation of your health. Everyone deserves a better life far from the specter of chronic disease and universal precautions, don't they? You can put on a happy face for your children, but if you're just starting a relationship with someone, you may harbor rather unusual, ambiguous feelings that are quite impossible to describe to someone who doesn't have a chronic diagnosis.

"I was worried that my husband wouldn't want to be involved with someone who is 'damaged,'" says Iris, "and now, if we argue and I make him mad, I think I'd better back down or he'll go find someone nicer and healthier. But I know he really loves me because it doesn't matter that I have HBV to him, and in a way it seems that I am more precious to him because he never takes for granted that I will always be around."

These may sound like gloomy sentiments, but HBV makes us experience a knee-jerk reaction that has us pushing away those we love most in order to save them from misery. We sometimes project a vision of our potential partner's suffering onto some worst-case future scenario. Our intentions are good, but we will also very likely have to deal with the possibility that our partner will question and distrust our real intent. How could anyone understand why you want to push them away unless you don't love them anymore? HBV may make you feel like you are bad news, as if you had big scarlet HBV letters sewn on your shirt.

It is difficult to let people take responsibility for choosing their future with us. But thankfully, sometimes people love us for who we are, regardless of our HBV status.

I'm afraid of getting/giving it

Some people avoid us like the plague, even if they can take steps to avoid contagion.

Bob is a 38-year-old teacher: "Hep B has affected my relationships. I'm single, and have dated a few nice ladies over the years, but now I have to accept that my body is contaminated. The last lady I dated didn't want to risk even safe sex with me. She was a widow and all her kids had in the world. It was only at that moment that I realized my circumstances had changed. This disease must now be factored into everything. Before her, all this was just academics to me: surface antigens, ALT levels, core antibodies—as a teacher I enjoy academic matters. But it's not academic anymore."

Unlike HIV, herpes, or sexually transmitted diseases, there is an effective vaccine against HBV. The first shot in the series provides a significant level of protection, although it is always a good idea to practice safe sex. If you are seeing someone who is still in a panic after learning about the vaccine's efficacy, there is little you can do except lay out the facts clearly. Sometimes even those who have already received the vaccine can be skittish about having sex. Show them HBV websites, CDC documents, or fliers from your local clinic to back up the information you've already provided. If all else fails, try a joint visit to a doctor or even a therapist.

Self image—hepper rhymes with leper

Many people use the term hepper to describe those who have joined the HBV club. I find the term unbearable because it rhymes with leper and emphasizes the ostracism we experience daily. Whatever we choose to call ourselves, there's no denying that we've been inducted into something against our will. It's a good idea to decide to make the best of it. After love and war, little bonds people so thoroughly and steadfastly as solidarity against a disease and the suffering it can cause.

It's all too natural and all too easy to let HBV drag down your self-esteem. When you let yourself go down that road, remember that you'll eventually come to a crossroads that offers the choice of either a positive or negative turn. Don't forget that you're in the driver's seat. The negative turn may seem like a short cut, but the positive turn is a more scenic route and it's the higher road. Every day, you have the freedom to choose the road you want to go down.

Be careful not to push your partner into a subordinate role

Some of us are blessed with partners who love us no matter what happens to our livers. They happily adapt their diets to ours, they don't make a face when we whine, and they happily rent a movie when we don't feel well enough to go out to a theater. They make love to us despite the presence of the virus. Would we do that if we were in their shoes? It's a healthy question to ask, and it keeps us mindful of what they must be experiencing as they care for our bodies and minds.

We may appreciate their help so much that we coin a term of endearment for this role they've selflessly agreed to take on. This is all well and good but it can hide potentially harmful aspects. Pam is wise to point them out: "I detest the phrase hepper helper! It implies that the focus of the universe is the person living with hep and all others are peripheral. I agree that the person living with hep should be the focus of their own universe, at least until they have their life in balance. But it is not OK in my opinion for others to be defined in that way. If I have a role, it is a friend, partner, lover, or whatever, but not a helper! I'm no Boy Scout and I'm not a servant (particularly if I'm not paid)! It is as irritating a phrase as 'consumer.' "

Chronic disease can be a magnet for codependency. Avoid allowing HBV to create a dynamic in which your relationship becomes lopsided and in which resentment gradually builds.

IN A SENTENCE:

Although there are considerations and precautions, you can still be intimate and enjoy a normal sex life with HBV.

learning

Charting your HBV

Charting can help both you and your doctor

I HAD a visit with my physician recently. They couldn't find my chart, so we just did without. No big deal, right? It is the third time it has happened to me (with 3 different doctors). I keep my own chart now, so I wasn't too concerned. But what if I hadn't been to this doctor in months? What if he has so many patients he couldn't remember me? What if I couldn't understand the difference between HBsAg and Anti-HBc? At a very minimum, it would have been a waste of my time. At the worst, I could have received a lazy diagnosis of hepatitis C, something that actually happened to me when my chart had been lost soon after my diagnosis many years ago.

If you haven't been charting your own lab tests or keeping copies of all of your labs, the news that your chart is missing can make you nervous, if not outright irritated. Given that so many people may need to consult the chart (biller, appointment scheduler, doctor, phlebotomist, nurse) and that you probably have appointments every few months, it is wise to make sure you have a second chart at home in a safe place.

Charting your ALT and AST is useful and wise

After your doctor's visit, ask the nurse for copies of any test results that may have been discussed with the doctor. Let them know that you're keeping your own files and don't want to lose the papers, and wait until they bring the copies. If a copier isn't available, jot down the test results in your notebook. I even bought a blank patient chart with tabs from a medical supply company so that I could keep the tests and doctor's notes the same way they do. My chart was lost for over 6 months a few years ago, so my homemade chart was a lifesaver.

If you've been doing regular blood work over the past months or years, try charting the material in a graph. Pam jokingly calls this hepnosis. Use the chart function in Excel, PowerPoint, or other spreadsheet program to graph your ALT and AST. This is something that software could easily accomplish for doctors if hospitals and clinics were more on the cutting edge of technology, and probably in the next few years we will see a marked increase in medical software systems geared to tracking and monitoring of treatment, tests, and medication. In the meantime, you can use this low-tech method to paint an objective, clear portrait of the ebb and flow of your enzymes if you prepare a simple chart. Ask a friend to help you if you aren't computer literate. Make sure you chart not only the enzyme levels on the vertical axis, but also the date of the test on the horizontal axis. And use separate colors for each line.

For a low-tech version of tracking, you can create a spreadsheet on a piece of graph paper or create your own grid. You lab test names go on the left-hand column and your scores on the horizontal lines you've drawn. You can still track your blood work even without a computer. See Resources for a complete tracking chart. Here is an abridged example:

	1/99	6/99	2/00	6/00	1/01	5/01	2/02	9/02	2/03
ALT	180	160	100	140	70	50	26		
AST	160	170	110	120	60	70	40		
DNA	5.7M	2.5M	100K	40K	2500	1100	500		

Often people who are just getting a handle on HBV have to call their doctors frequently to figure out what tests have been performed or not, and most often a nurse will return calls. A lot of confusion can take place when trying to get answers over the phone. Keeping your own chart will also make it helpful for your support group to assist you with treatment decisions or other HBV issues. We don't have to be obsessive about tracking, but it is a good way to stay just that: on track. To others who don't have a disease it may be perceived as a neurotic and self-indulgent exercise, and some doctors are suspicious of patients who come too prepared and are too focused on their ailment. Don't worry about what others think.

Charting helps you stay in control of your treatment

It's easier to know if you're with the right doctor if you keep track of your chart. Hepatitis is confusing for everyone. But it is especially tough for those who have just been diagnosed, and a new diagnosis is a time when critical decisions need to be made. If you suspect that your doctor or specialist isn't very well prepared to care for you, you will have a much easier time finding objective answers about what to do if you have all of your tests on hand, or find a new doctor.

Even if you have the best hepatologist in your area, charting helps you feel like you aren't going crazy. With all of its intricate logic, HBV can test your patience. Maureen has become one of the most informed people on earth about HBV, and she can still get frustrated: "It seems like every step I take forward I take two steps backward with my knowledge of HBV. Everything I learn and read is refuted somewhere else. I feel the need to consult at least three specialists to see if I might possibly be able to gain a consensus. So far that's not working. Everybody has a different opinion, or they just clam up."

Charting also helps you be prepared for benefits paperwork, and it is essential if you think you might qualify for Social Security benefits or disability payments. See Month 6 for an in-depth discussion about Social Security benefits and disability.

Charting your mood can be helpful if you have periods of depression

Charting and journaling can save your life. Interferon treatment can induce severe depression, so it's not a bad idea to prepare for a worst-case scenario by charting your mood in the weeks *before* you start treatment. Although you should have already informed your family and closest friends about likely side effects, you can often be sucked into a kind of mood blind spot when you're on treatment, forgetting that your depression is chemically induced. Give your mood a point score of 1–10 every day before you go to bed, and let your doctor and loved ones know when your score is low for more than a few days.

Your stools may reflect how your liver is doing

One of the quickest ways of gauging how your gastrointestinal system is doing is by glancing at your bowel movements. Information about unusual size, shape, color, and consistency can be useful for your doctor, in addition to changes in frequency. Keeping accurate information can be valuable especially if you are experiencing cramps or other abdominal distress or pain.

You may think that it is a bit excessive to track these changes, but you don't have to keep a chart next to the toilet. However, it is wise to be mindful, especially if you have changed your diet or are going through a particularly stressful period. Make at least a mental note of any medications or herbs you're taking, or any antacids or laxatives. If your stools are either too dry or too watery for long periods, you should mention it to your doctor. Thin strands of stool seen over an extended period are also something you should mention to your doctor, as you could be experiencing blockage in the colon or parasites.

Vegetarians in general have lighter stools, while those who eat meat or take antacids or iron supplements have dark stools. Call your doctor if you notice very dark, tarry stools, as this may mean that bleeding is occurring somewhere in your digestive tract. Light or clay-colored stools are not unusual to see in people who have HBV and cirrhosis, and may point to an obstruction of bile flow from the liver or a lack of bile salt production.

IN A SENTENCE:

> Charting your labs, diet, and fatigue will give you a more objective view of your hepatitis, and it give you an extra tool to help your doctor.

Become an HBV Activist

Grassroots: YOU are the media

THE INTERNET allows us to reach others halfway around the world and virtually welcome people into our minds, hearts, and homes. Now we can send e-mails to hundreds of politicians and journalists at the click of a mouse, or take advantage of databases for digital grassroots initiatives. I'm happy to report that there is already an active and supportive online HBV world, and you can look into it when you like. However, not enough information is available yet to those who are still susceptible to HBV. In our own way, we can all be proactive in this regard. Here are a few examples and opportunities.

The Hepatitis B Foundation

The Hepatitis B Foundation (HBF) is the only national non-profit organization dedicated solely to the cause and cure of hepatitis B. It is a wonderful group of caring, committed individuals who sincerely seek to help improve the quality of life for all those affected by chronic hepatitis B through research, education, and patient support. I love the HBF because they are 100 percent geared towards helping people like you and me.

The HBF was founded in 1991 by two couples, Paul and Janine Witte and Tim and Joan Block, who responded to the plight of a young family suffering from hepatitis B. When they discovered there was no organization that could provide information or support, they decided to establish the HBF to help others and to ensure that there was a focused effort to fund research to find a cure. They have since grown from a local grassroots effort into a substantial organization with a global reach.

Thousands of people with HBV are assisted via phone, e-mail and snail mail. The HBF offers a comprehensive and multilingual website and a highly responsive and personal e-mail service and phone help line, which is answered by a knowledgeable live person. They also have a thorough range of free literature, and their *B-Informed* newsletter is one of the only free newsletters available. Be sure to ask for it, as it contains a useful HBV Drug Watch section with a rundown of the latest treatment developments.

The HBF's research laboratory at Jefferson Medical College is the site of the exciting discovery of a plant sugar-derived HBV antiviral compound that is expected to go into human trials late this year. See Month 7 for a discussion of their imino sugars research. The HBF also sponsors the prestigious annual Princeton Workshop where a small group of the nation's leading researchers and clinical experts are invited to come together to discuss HBV therapeutics. The first ever HBV patient conference was organized by the HBF last year, and was an overwhelming success. Call them for information on the next conference.

In addition, the foundation testifies before state and national legislatures on behalf of the millions of HBV-infected individuals and families and remains at the forefront towards establishing a research agenda for finding a cure.

Like all nonprofit groups, the HBF depends on your generosity. Call them today to see how you can help. Giving hope to millions is as easy as giving a donation.

Latino Organization for Liver Awareness (LOLA)

An enterprising transplant recipient named Debbie Delgado-Vega founded the Latino Organization for Liver Awareness (LOLA). In 1994, Debbie's liver decompensated rapidly due to a severe case of autoimmune hepatitis. She was lucky enough to receive a liver just in time, and the experience led her to dedicate her life to creating the first bilingual liver resource/referral center in the nation. LOLA's goal is to promote organ donation among Latino communities throughout the United States.

LOLA, a voluntary and entirely bilingual and bicultural organization, is also dedicated to raising awareness, prevention, education, and treatment referral services to the Latino community and other underserved populations who suffer from liver disease in the United States. Despite the boom of resources on the Internet, only a small percentage is presented in a bilingual format. LOLA sometimes hosts benefits to pay tribute to donor families, transplant patients and transplant professionals who have given of themselves to further the cause of organ donation and transplantation in New York's Latino community area. They also organize frequent support group meetings out of the New York Blood Center (see below).

LOLA is a nonprofit organization supported by grants, private and corporate contributions, fund-raising events, and individuals like you.

Awareness among Asians and Pacific Islanders

Asians have the highest rate of hepatitis B of all ethnic groups. Seventy-five percent of those with chronic HBV worldwide (about 260 million) reside in Asia. And 80 percent of liver cancer in Asian Americans is caused by chronic hepatitis B virus infection. Chinese authorities recently reported that two thirds of China's population has been infected with hepatitis B. Reuse of syringes, a common practice in China, is a leading factor of this ominous statistic. Over 300,000 Chinese die of HBV-related liver cancer and cirrhosis annually.

On this side of the ocean, the nonprofit Asian Liver Center of Stanford University organized the Jade Ribbon Campaign to increase awareness and provide ethnic-sensitive health information to the API (Asian and Pacific Islander) community and health professionals. The Asian Liver Center is a clinical resource center for the public and health care professionals, and it spearheads efforts to formulate public health care policies and seek grants to address the needs of the Asian-American community. The center also develops clinical and basic research programs. You can request materials in Korean, Chinese, Vietnamese, or English, or make a donation by calling (650) 72-LIVER. Or visit their informative website http://livercancer.stanford.edu/index.asp or http://liver.stanford.edu.

The Hepatitis B Foundation offers a Chinese version of their website. Go to www.hepb.org/c/.

You can also call GlaxoSmithKline's HBV Information and Assistance Line for the Asian community. They provide physician referrals and screening sites, and provide their service in Mandarin, Cantonese, Korean, Vietnamese, and English. Call (888) 888-0981.

Web activism: all you need is a computer

www.Congress.org is a quick reference guide to your elected officials. Or check out www.HepatitisActivist.org, which has an automatic e-mail generator on topics such as: increasing government research funding for liver diseases and education initiatives, transplant program improvement, FDA fast-track approval for promising new drugs, Social Security/insurance/disability reform, and veterans' issues. Although most of the letters refer to HCV, you can cut and paste the sample letters and adapt them to your needs.

You can volunteer for foundation events

Check with your local American Liver Foundation (ALF) office for information about local fund-raising drives or informational seminars. The ALF sponsors countless walks, runs, and seminars across the country. Go to www.liverfoundation.org or call them at 1-800-GOLIVER. The Hepatitis B Foundation also organizes fund-raising events, like the annual HBF Crystal Ball. Contact them for more information.

Hepatitis B Foundation
700 East Butler Avenue
Doylestown, PA 18901
(215) 489-4900

Latino Organization for Liver Awareness (LOLA)
Debbie Delgado-Vega, Founder and CEO
P.O. Box 842
Throggs Neck Station
Bronx, New York 10465
(718) 892-8697 Phone
1-888-367-LOLA (Toll Free)
www.lola-national.org/

New York Blood Center
310 East 67th Street
New York, NY 10021
(212) 570-3010

IN A SENTENCE:

> *You can get the word out about HBV and help save lives.*

Mutants

MUTANT HBV sounds like something out of a bad science fiction movie, and the term may be somewhat misleading. Mutations are occurring naturally in our bodies and in nature. The significance of mutants varies, however. Some go unnoticed, some cannot reproduce, and others may be successful at surviving but aren't as virulent. In other words, you shouldn't feel anxious or scared when you hear the term.

There are two types of mutations: one develops as an offensive action against a drug (known as drug-resistance), and the others occur naturally and spontaneously as a variation on a theme. When you hear your doctor or support group members refer to the wild-type virus, they are talking about the virus that grows wild in your liver, not the mutant. In general, mutant HBV is less virulent and thus less harmful than wild-type HBV. But if you have more than one type of mutant HBV in your system or significant amounts of any variety of HBV in your blood, HBV can still do harm. And sometimes mutants can pass undetected in tests.

What exactly is a mutant?

As we learned in Day 3, the hepatitis B virus consists of a surface and a core, and there are S (surface), C (core), and e antigen/antibody groups. When we want to dig a little deeper into HBV's personality and its defense mechanisms, we need look at the various components of these various antigens. The S antigen, for example, can be further divided into different components called regions, and these are known as pre-S1 and pre-S2. It is quite rare for a mutation to occur with the S antigen, but if this happens a person may test negative for the S antigen but still have detectable HBV DNA in his blood. Infants or people with weak immune systems who receive HBiG or the HBV vaccine may also develop HBV surface gene mutations. The mutants are usually no longer detectable in blood unless HBV DNA and e antigen tests are carried out. And sometimes we can't even determine which mutant is present because there aren't yet standardized lab tests available outside of academic research labs.

Likewise, the core antigen is divided into two regions, the pre-core and the core. It does have a greater propensity to mutate, so what we sometimes find is that some people are S positive, HBV DNA positive, but e antigen negative. The pre-core mutant is more common in Southern Europe, Asia, Africa, the Middle East, and the Mediterranean.

People taking Lamivudine may develop a **YMDD** mutation involving the DNA polymerase after 6 months or more of treatment with the drug.

If this wasn't sufficiently complex, HBsAg particles can be further broken down into subgroups: adw, adr, ayw, and ayr. Maureen invented a great metaphor to describe HBV mutations: "Think of HBV's DNA as a zipper. On each side of the zipper are little teeth. When you zip up, you might not always match the one side of the zipper with the other side. Just having one tooth of the zipper out of synch is a mutation. Some are more successful and aggressive, and others are not successful and can't replicate."

Be on the lookout for mutants

Now that you've probably been on either Lamivudine or Interferon, it is important to know about these mutations so that you can be on the lookout for their appearance. You may have charted a significant decrease in your viral load over the past 3 months. Mine, for example, went from 5.7 million to 200 in just a few months. In fact, you may even continue to see very low or undetectable HBV DNA in your blood for years. But if you see a spike while you are still on a medication, you may be witnessing the birth of a mutant strain. It's good to manage your expectations about this possibility and be prepared if this happens to you. If it does, it usually means that it is time to rethink your treatment strategy or dosage.

Adefovir may be effective against mutant HBV

Those of us who have been taking Lamivudine for more than a year start wondering if we will develop resistance to the drug. While the longer you take Lamivudine the greater your chance of mutation, new drugs like Adefovir and Entecavir may eliminate even these mutations. It is not known, however, if resistance will eventually develop against these drugs as well. Time will only tell. Adefovir does not promote the development of YMDD variants and apparently is effective in treating YMDD variants that have developed in patients who have received Lamivudine. Whether Adefovir should be alone or in combination with Lamivudine remains to be determined.

Trials have shown that Entecavir is also active against Lamivudine-resistant HBV variants and in those people who have not seen improvement from Lamivudine. Further studies on dosage and length of treatment are now being carried out, as well as studies on its safety.

IN A SENTENCE:

> *Mutants are due to either drug resistance or natural causes, but it is best to be informed about them so you know what to do if and when they appear in your bloodstream.*

living

Having/Raising/
Adopting Children

IT IS thought that as many as 5 percent of adopted Asian children are HBV carriers. Even if infants are tested at birth, some medical professionals ignore test reports conducted in Asia because the children may be too young to demonstrate infection or because they do not trust foreign testing methods. Some countries avoid testing altogether due to a lack of clean needles, and they may understandably feel that children who are diagnosed may not find a home. If you or friends are considering adopting in Asia and do not have HBV, it may be wise to start the vaccine series before going. Even if your adopted child tested negative before joining your family, he or she may have been subsequently infected in the orphanage, clinic, or through testing with infected needles or other medical instruments. For this reason it is wise to retest after six months.

Teach your children about universal precautions

In a mixed household—a home where both HBV and non-HBV people live—it is important to practice universal precautions. Children are effective transmitters of HBV given that they play hard, tend to have more accidents involving blood, and generally are a little freer with their DNA than adults. If you have HBV and your child doesn't, it is wise to place razors, brushes, nail clippers, and other items that may contain traces of your blood out of reach. Talk to your children about the importance of not touching other people's blood. After all, those with HBV are also at risk for acquiring other infectious diseases.

Newborns can be protected against infection from HBV+ mothers

Hepatitis B does not usually affect the health of an unborn baby. But pregnant women who are infected with HBV can transmit the virus to their newborns during the delivery process. For this reason, it is essential that all women be tested for HBV, and ideally all newborns should be vaccinated within 12 hours of birth to protect them from chronic infection. If you have HBV, remind the doctor who will be delivering your child to order the hepatitis B vaccine and one dose of HBiG (hepatitis B immunoglobulin), and tell the doctor that you want this vaccine and HBiG to be administered in the delivery room. It's a good idea to remind your partner to make sure this is done since you may very well be too tired to ask. Unfortunately, if the vaccine is incorrectly administered, your baby will most likely become chronically infected with HBV.

More than 90 percent of pregnant women with HBV pass the virus on to their newborn. This is called **perinatal transmission**. Infants of infected mothers should receive both HBIG (hepatitis B immune globulin) and the first HBV vaccine shot. In most cases this procedure protects the infant from HBV.

Breastfeeding is safe unless there is bleeding or discharge from the nipples or evidence of **mastitis**. Both the CDC and WHO strongly encourage women to breastfeed.

Telling the school

If your state requires HBV vaccinations, you will need to have your doctor handle paperwork for your child. See Day 3 for more about your rights when disclosing your child's HBV status to the school.

There are numerous emotional issues for children and teens

Avoiding alcohol and finding a partner are hard enough as an adult, so imagine how difficult it must be for someone with HBV who is already trying to deal with high school, acne, peer pressure to try drugs or alcohol, stress, and doubts about the future. And, although children and teens with HBV need extra understanding and support, it may take practice for parents to balance equal amounts of love and emotional support among other, noninfected children. It's a good idea to encourage brothers and sisters to provide some of that support so that there is horizontal distribution in the family.

Unlike diseases that are visible, HBV presents a special problem. As an invisible illness, too much prevention, apprehension, and consideration may feel exaggerated to your children, friends, schoolmates, and neighbors, while not enough may seem almost callous. It's a good idea to encourage a teen with HBV to get involved in a support group like the online HBV listserv. And joining the Parents of Kids with Infectious Diseases (PKIDs) group (www.pkids.org/listserv.htm) will help you gain a basic understanding of the various issues parents face.

Parents can feel guilty about infecting their children

Kirstin has experienced the full range of feelings about being a HBV parent with an HBV child: "I feel guilt every day when I look at my son, see a hep commercial and especially around other kids in our extended family. I know their parents fear me touching them, so I don't. Most of the time I remain at a distance. They are afraid of my son touching their toys, to change his diaper . . . and even when he spits up. They have even gone as far as to put rubber gloves in his diaper bag with no explanation."

HBV children of HBV parents also feel guilty about discussing their illness with their parents, especially if they inherited the virus from them. "I don't share bad labs or biopsy results with my mother, because I know it makes her feel guilty even though HBV isn't her fault," says Iris, "I also don't discuss my HBV with her because she doesn't understand why I'm always trying to study the latest treatments and developments. She never did any treatment and she's 'just fine,' so why aren't we."

Minimize the risk of spreading infection

Wear gloves when cleaning up blood or other bodily fluids. A diluted bleach solution (one part bleach to nine parts water or stronger) will kill the virus. Clothing with bloodstains should also be washed in a diluted solution of bleach. Household alcohol, such as rubbing alcohol, will also kill the virus. Dispose of your cleaning materials safely, and thoroughly wash your hands afterwards.

Contact PKIDs for more information and support

PKIDs (Parents of Kids with Infectious Diseases) is a national nonprofit organization founded in 1996 after a few parents had difficulty finding baby-sitters or playmates willing to spend time with their infected children, and the organization is the first of its kind. PKIDs' mission is to "educate the public about infectious diseases, the methods of prevention and transmission, the latest advances in medicine, and the elimination of social stigma borne by the infected; and to assist the families of the children living with hepatitis, HIV/AIDS, or other chronic, viral infectious diseases with emotional, financial, and informational support."

There is also an unmoderated "Parent Support Email Community" listserv. Here, parents of children with HBV, HCV, HIV, and other infectious diseases can find support and community. The PKIDs site describes this forum as a place where parents can "exchange information about medical issues and treatments, problems of discrimination, who to tell and how to talk to our children. Essentially, this is a great place to vent, rejoice, and get help when you need it." You can join the list by going to their listserv subscription page at www.pkids.org/listserv.htm, visit their home page: www.pkids.org, or call toll free: (877) 55-PKIDS.

Comeunity is a useful resource for adoptive parents

Comeunity is a not for profit, volunteer website with the goal of benefiting children by building diverse communities and providing family centered support. The site provides high quality information in a supportive atmosphere and serves multiple communities in the adoption and special needs arena. You can find professional and parent-authored articles, newsletters, mailing lists, and resources that help parents provide the best care for their children. You can log on at www.comeunity.com/index.html, or go directly to their comprehensive HBV pages at www.comeunity.com/adoption/health/hepatitis/index.html.

Join a parents support group

You can also join an online support group for parents of adopted children with HBV. The HBV Adoption Listserv Support Group can be found at www.onelist.com/subscribe/hbv-adoption, or contact Bambi Winkler at bambi@americansisp.com.

IN A SENTENCE:

> *There are many special medical, emotional, and social considerations when the person with HBV is a child, so it is important to reach out to other parents who can identify with what you're experiencing.*

learning

Treatment Issues for Children

IN DAY 5 we discussed how important it is to keep your primary physician, even though you will be going to your hepatologist for all liver-related issues. Just as your own primary physician should be part of your team, your child's pediatrician should be thought of as a case manager who can oversee the big picture of your child's health. Ideally, the pediatrician will be interested in helping interpret lab tests and answering basic questions, but hopefully he or she will also defer to the hepatologist on more difficult issues. Avoid letting the pediatrician take over full responsibility for your child's case, unless, of course, they have extensive experience in hepatology.

Lab results know something about Murphy's Law

Once you are fully informed about the different lab tests that will be run, you can ask to check the lab orders before any blood is drawn. This will minimize administrative errors or oversights. Very often the wrong boxes are checked, wrong tests ordered, or the tests are repeated unnecessarily. This is hard for anyone, but especially difficult for young children. You can also make sure that the doctor looks over the sheet before the draw.

When you're trying to manage two or more doctors at the same time, you should choose to send the labs to one or the other, as many labs have automated their reporting system so much that only one fax number is allowed. Sometimes your labs drop into a big black hole, never to be found again by anyone. That has happened to me. It's particularly distressing when it is your child that has to go back for another draw. If this happens, make sure the second draw and test aren't charged. There is no need to get really upset, but let the doctor and his office know that you are in control.

Again, insist on receiving copies of all labs before you leave the office. Lab results seem to follow Murphy's Law to the last clause: if they can be lost, they will be lost.

You can help make testing easier on your child

Biopsies. Absolutely no movement can occur during the actual biopsy, so if your child is very young or prone to agitation in clinical settings, discuss what kind of conscious sedation or anesthetic might be used. Try to schedule the procedure as early as possible, so your child won't have to fast too long. And, since your child is fasting, avoid eating or drinking in his or her presence. Take a stuffed animal, favorite book, and a stroller to the hospital—it will comfort your child and provide a familiar setting.

Interferon injections. If possible, dedicate a room in your home to the shots. This will help to instill confidence and trust. Don't try to use the kitchen or bathroom, as they may be the least hygienic. Practice a system in tandem so that the shot can be carried out quickly, since anticipation of the shot is usually worse than reality. Maureen has a good system worked out: "We did the shots right before her bath. One of us would go up to prepare the injections and alcohol wipe, while the other would come up baring her leg for the injection. That way less than 30 seconds passed from start to finish, and her tears were gone in less than a minute." Liz was pleasantly surprised at how involved her daughter became in her treatment: "We were stunned when my daughter was diagnosed with HBV. She didn't fit our picture of someone with active hepatitis. My daughter has done exceptionally well on Interferon. I am not having the best time with it from a parent's perspective, but we are getting through it. It has lowered her viral load to nondetectable and her liver functions to normal. She even helps out with her shots."

Blood tests. Make sure that your child is well-hydrated before the blood draw, especially if your child's veins are hard to locate. Excess fluids will help the veins be more visible. If you or your child likes one phlebotomist in particular, try to have the same one do the draws each time.

Call ahead to make sure the staff member you want is in the office. A good phlebotomist knows that quick handling of the vials and needles mitigates much of the anxiety we feel about having blood drawn. It doesn't hurt to request that they prepare all of the vials in advance so that no time is wasted with the child present. If your child is prone to fainting or being ill during draws, you can talk to your doctor about the possibility of having your child take a mild sedative before you get to the doctor's office.

More inexperienced doctors may resist treating your child's HBV

You may find that doctors that treat adults may choose not to treat your child, even if he or she meets all the criteria for treatment. No one likes to see a child suffer, so you may need to find a pediatric specialist who has sufficient experience and who will treat the needs of your child at this critical time.

IN A SENTENCE:

HBV acts quite differently in children, so find a pediatric hepatologist or GI specialist who has experience with juvenile HBV.

MONTH **6**

living

Work
and Disability

"HERE'S THE brutal truth about disability: they don't
want to give it to you. It's a process fraught with hurdles, aimed
at getting you to go away," says Ed Mahoney. Disability is sup-
posed to be a kind of safety net for when we're unable to work.
That's partially why we pay taxes. Many of us with fibrosis and
cirrhosis have a tough enough time getting out of bed, let alone
bringing home the bacon. Often, even if we have the energy to
complete our tasks, we have brain fog to deal with. The following are the many and complicated steps that you must take
if you think you might qualify for long-term disability payments.

The Social Security Administration has two programs: the
Social Security disability insurance program and the Supplemental Security Income (SSI) program. Eligibility for Social
Security disability is based on contributions you made through
your previous employers, where you contributed to your own
Social Security account; SSI disability payments are based of
financial need.

There are other differences in the eligibility rules for the two
programs. The Social Security Administration has a booklet
dealing primarily with the Social Security disability insurance
program. You can stop by any Social Security office and ask for
the booklet (SSI publication no. 05-11000). You can also obtain

this information online by going to: http://www.ssa.gov/pubs/11000.html. Questions can also be answered by calling the Social Security Administration's toll-free number at (800) 772-1213, but be prepared for a lengthy wait.

When you begin the application process, bear in mind that each application is reviewed on a case-by-case basis. Don't be discouraged because someone else with hepatitis has been turned down. Many factors can affect the Administration's decision including, but not limited to, your specific impairments, education, age, and supporting medical evidence to substantiate your claim.

The following are five considerations that may help you determine if you qualify for disability benefits:

1. You are working but earn less than $500 a month.
2. Your disability interferes with basic work-related activities.
3. Your disability is on the Social Security Administration's "List of Impairments" or your documentation, including your medical history, proves that your condition is of equal severity to others on the list.
4. Your condition interferes with your ability to perform jobs you've had within the last 15 years.
5. Your condition prevents you from performing tasks that are appropriate for your age, education, experience, skills, and demands.

Remember to provide complete documentation and to keep copies for yourself.

You must have already left your job

Although it may sound peculiar, for the government you must have already left your job because of your disability. There is a five-month waiting period before you can receive your first check if your application is approved. If you attempt to work during this five-month period, Social Security will consider you ineligible because you are able to work. Before leaving your job, you may want to do a little investigating into what kind of monthly payment you can expect from the government, as you may be quite disappointed at how little it may be.

You must fill out a ton of forms

Although many people believe that you initiate the process through your doctor, you can also begin the process on your own. After your initial inquiry, you will receive an application from Social Security asking about your daily activities and what you can and cannot do physically. You should fill this out as if it were your worst day. In the meantime, Social Security will request all of your medical records. You simply provide the names and addresses of your doctors and they do the rest. If you haven't already, get copies of all of your lab tests, doctors notes, biopsy reports, and other medical documents for your own records. You will need them.

In the meantime, read the liver section in your Social Security "Listing of Impairments" to look at what is required to qualify for benefits. For hepatitis B, you will have to have experienced documented esophageal varices and/or performance of a shunt operation to repair them, bilirubin of 2.5 mg per deciliter or greater persisting for at least five months, ascites due to HBV persisting for at least five months, and/or hepatic encephalopathy. In addition, you should have confirmation of chronic liver disease by biopsy and one of the following: recurring ascites, bilirubin of 2.5 per deciliter for at least three months, or hepatic cell necrosis or inflammation for a least three months with elevated enzymes.

Making the call

Once you've reviewed the listing and can determine that you qualify, you can write a letter to your Social Security caseworker (the name will be printed on everything you receive from the Social Security office) stating that you qualify for a listing and include copies of your medical records that prove your claim. If you don't qualify for a listing you will obviously be turned down. This doesn't mean that you can't get disability, but that the process moves into an area of subjective determination. The caseworker will try to determine if you are able to carry out any of the jobs you've done in the past ten years. They will not take into consideration if you can live off that salary or not.

Avoid dropping down to part-time work

If you can afford it or can do work from home, it may seem like a good idea to work part-time, especially if you can keep your benefits. This can be a bad idea, especially if you are planning to apply for disability. Although it may seem like a reasonable thing to do, the government doesn't think so. You will be penalized for working part-time if and when it comes to calculating your monthly Social Security payments.

Hire a lawyer if you are turned down and think you have the right to benefits

Roughly 80–90 percent of all Social Security applications are turned down during the first round. This may be due, in part, to the fact that forms are incomplete or have been filled out incorrectly by you or your physician. A careful review of forms is a good idea before you send them off. It may be necessary for your doctor to write a follow-up letter with detailed justification for your disability. If you are denied benefits and you believe that you have a right to them based on your medical records, hire a lawyer as soon as you can. There are strict deadlines for completing the appeal process—for instance, you have 60 days from the time you receive the letter from the Social Security Administration to file an appeal. The Administration assumes you received their letter with the denial decision five days after the date on it, unless you can prove that you received it later. The lawyer will be paid a fixed percentage (currently 25 percent of your back payments starting after 5 months from your last day of work). Although 80–90 percent of applicants are turned down during the appeal process, your lawyer can file to be heard before a judge. This process can take quite a long time, and you must remember that you must not work during this process or you will disqualify yourself.

If the judge sides with you and awards you benefits, you do not automatically qualify for Medicare benefits, as there is a two-year waiting period after the first five months. Like it or not, you will have to wait another two years before you can qualify for Medicare.

IN A SENTENCE:

> *Disability payments may be available if you qualify, but if you think you might apply, there are lengthy procedures to follow and documentation to gather.*

Insurance and Financial Planning

INSURANCE IS defined as coverage by contract whereby one party undertakes to indemnify or guarantee another against loss by a specified contingency or peril. For our purposes, this would be a health insurer protecting you from financial loss.

In the United States, many individuals obtain medical coverage for themselves and their families through their employers. Benefits are generally provided after a specified length of time at your job (usually one month although there are cases where coverage begins immediately). Obvious exceptions are individuals who are self-employed and require their own private health insurance, or those in a high-risk pool.

There are different types of insurance

There are two types of health insurance: fee-for-service (indemnity) and managed care. Both have a basic premium, although how much your employer pays and how much you pay varies by plan and employer. It is your responsibility to research the plans and determine which type is best for you. Reading the fine print is particularly important if you or someone covered under your plan has a potentially serious or chronic medical condition.

There are many differences between health insurance plans. Deciding which plan is best for you can be pretty confusing. The easiest way to break it down is by asking yourself the following: Is going to a doctor of my choice the single most important factor? If you answer yes, an indemnity plan is probably the way to go. If you don't mind choosing from a preselected list of doctors, which may or may not include the family doctor you've been going to for years, and if you don't mind traveling to a new office, then a managed care program may be right for you. The trade-off to not having the freedom to choose your doctor is the potential of reduced cost of services (e.g., lower copay or deductible), less paperwork, and lower out-of-pocket expenses for you.

If you determine that a managed health care plan is right for you, the next step is deciding which type of network best suits your needs.

Managed health care plans

There are three major managed care plans to choose from: Preferred Provider Organization (PPO), Health Maintenance Organization (HMO), and POS (Point-of-Service).

A PPO is an organization providing health care that provides economic incentives to the individual purchaser of a health care contract. In order to optimize your benefits, you are asked to patronize certain physicians, laboratories, and hospitals that agree to supervision and reduced fees. The network providers have prearranged contracts with your PPO to accept lower fees in exchange for their services. In theory, your portion of the cost of services is lowered. PPOs also allow you to step out-of-network and see the caregiver of your choice. This would result in higher out-of-pocket expenses for you, so you are encouraged to stay within the network. The most appealing aspect of this plan is the freedom to choose your provider.

An HMO is an organization that provides comprehensive health care to voluntarily enrolled individuals and families. Members are usually limited to a particular geographic area and member physicians have limited referral to outside specialists. Like PPOs, HMOs are financed by fixed periodic payments determined in advance through prearranged contracts. Copayments are predetermined and generally fairly minimal. There are no deductibles or claim forms when obtaining health care service.

A perceived drawback is the need to obtain referrals from your primary care physician (PCP) in order to visit a specialist. Although it seems counterintuitive to have your PCP provide a referral for an X ray deemed necessary by your dentist, it is how the program operates and you are penalized for not following the strict guidelines. The idea is that your PCP is responsible for your overall health care needs and is responsible for coordinating these efforts with other specialists within the network.

Another drawback to enrolling in an HMO is the total lack of freedom to choose any health care provider you want. You must choose from a list provided by the HMO. Any services you receive from providers outside of the network are entirely your financial responsibility.

The upside of an HMO is that they can be the least expensive health care alternative. Savings, of course, are determined by your general health and your health care needs.

POS is an alternative option provided by HMOs which allows you to stay within the network of providers, or you can be referred to an out-of-network provider. Generally, a network provider must obtain prior approval before referring you to an out-of-network provider. Justification for this referral is necessary before your HMO can cover all of the cost of services.

The bottom line is that you need to educate yourself on the differences in plans and make a decision about what is best for you. Employers have plan administrators in their Human Resources departments if you need or would like to have a professional help with your decision.

High-risk pools may help you afford insurance

According to the Health Care Financing Administration (HCFA), a high-risk pool is ". . . Any arrangement established and maintained by a State to provide health care insurance benefits to certain State residents who, because of their poor health history, are unable to purchase coverage in the open market or can only acquire such coverage at a rate that is substantially above the rate offered by the high-risk pool. Coverage offered by a high-risk pool is comparable to coverage available in the open market, but the risk for that coverage is borne by the State, which generally supports the losses sustained by the pool through assessments on all health insurers doing business in the State, based on their relative market share, and/or through general tax revenues."

Providing health care coverage through a high-risk pool is the government's way of ensuring that you are able to obtain some form of medical insurance benefits regardless of your state of health.

Uncle Sam can help (sometimes)

There are also some federally funded health care programs in place that can help. The two most prominent are Medicare and Medicaid. The U.S. Congress enacted them in 1965 as a means to provide individuals with health care alternatives. Medicare is a health insurance program for individuals 65 years of age and older, permanently disabled people under Social Security or Railroad Retirement programs, and persons of all ages with kidney disease (end stage renal disease, ESRD). I won't go into exhaustive detail about Medicare since it is a rather complicated program, but you do need to know that it exists as an alternative to group and individual health care plans.

One of the major drawbacks of Medicare is that it does not cover outpatient prescriptions. Since prescriptions are such an important part of any hepatitis treatment, it is often necessary to obtain supplemental insurance to fill in the holes. Medigap and Medicare SELECT are two plans you may want to look into. Medicaid is also an option for Medicare recipients who are in a low-income bracket. One thing you should be aware of is that Medicare does not cover most hepatitis treatments administered outside a physician's office. Therefore, self-administered injectables are not covered. You shouldn't feel discouraged, however, since Medicare programs are reviewing their prescription programs and injectable guidelines.

Medicaid is a program of medical aid designed for those unable to afford regular medical service and is financed by the state and federal governments. As a result of population gaps and varied state resources, Medicaid programs differ from state to state. Generally speaking, Medicaid covers hepatitis treatments in most states, but some programs are limited to the pharmacies located within the state. I can't emphasize enough how important it is to research and know what the program in your state covers.

Preexisting conditions

If you are currently uninsured and are diagnosed with hepatitis, it will be more difficult for you to obtain affordable insurance that will cover your medical needs. Most plans have preexisting clauses that allow the plan to exclude payment of your claims. The preexisting waiting period imposed by the clauses range between eight and twelve months. However, once the waiting period is over, your health plan is obligated to cover all of your future claims.

On the other hand, if you currently have health insurance and are switching jobs or plans, there is a federal law known as the Health Insurance Portability and Accountability Act (HIPAA) that protects patients from preexisting clauses. If you change insurance companies, it is the responsibility of the previous insurance to provide you with a Certificate of Portability. This certificate provides documented proof that you had prior insurance coverage. Your new insurance plan should honor your certificate by waiving any preexisting condition clauses.

Eligibility for HIPAA protection

According to the HCFA website, "If you are not currently covered by a particular type of plan or insurance, you need to determine what you may be eligible for.

1. Your eligibility to enroll in a group health plan is determined by the rules of the group health plan and the contract terms of any insurance purchased by an insured plan.
2. Your eligibility to have HIPAA guarantees you the right to purchase individual health insurance coverage (which, in some States, will be through a high-risk pool) depends on your ability to meet ALL of the following requirements:
    a. You have at least 18 months of creditable coverage without a significant break in coverage—a period of 63 days or more during all of which you had no coverage. If you get coverage by midnight of the 63rd day, you have not incurred a significant break;
    b. Your most recent coverage must have been through a health care group plan (through your or a family member's employer or union);
    c. You are not eligible for coverage under any group health plan;
    d. You are not eligible for Medicare or Medicaid;
    e. You do not have other health insurance;
    f. You did not lose your insurance for not paying the premiums or for committing fraud; and
    g. You accepted and used up your COBRA continuation coverage or similar State coverage if it was offered to you.

If you meet these requirements, you become a "HIPAA eligible individual."

For additional information on HIPAA and how it can protect you and your family, go to the HCFA website at www.hcfa.gov/medicaid/hipaa/content/hipsteps.asp.

No insurance? Want first dibs on a new drug? Look for a clinical trial

Clinical testing in the United States is usually done in three stages.

Phase I studies test the drug's safety among a small group of healthy volunteers. These participants are usually paid to take part. Phase I tests what happens to the body in the presence of the particular drug, and also determines what side effects take place as the dosage is gradually increased. You will probably not qualify for phase one studies, particularly if you have cirrhosis. Roughly 70 percent of drugs pass this phase.

Phase II tests the effectiveness of the given drug, and is for those who have the target condition or disease. This phase is usually randomized, meaning that some people receive the drug and some people receive a placebo, or sugar pill. Sometimes these trials are even blinded, meaning that neither the researcher nor patient knows who is receiving the actual drug. Only about 30 percent of drugs pass the first two hurdles.

Phase III is a large-scale test carried out in hundreds—even thousands—of people, and gives the FDA a better sense of the drug's effectiveness and side effects. Although this phase can last up to a few years, 70 to 90 percent of drugs pass Phase III testing and request FDA approval.

If you decide to participate in a study, you should ask a lot of questions. The last thing you need when your liver is already vulnerable is risk. Here are a few questions to direct to the research center:

O How long will the trial last?
O Is this a phase one or phase two trial?
O What kinds of tests will I have to undergo to qualify?
O Will I have to have another biopsy? More than one?
O How often will I have to go to be tested?
O What are the risks involved in the trial?
O What are the potential benefits of the drug being tested?
O Do I have to pay for anything?
O How many people will be participating in this study?
O Will I be paid for anything? (time off from work, transportation, etc.)
O What happens if the drug makes me sick?
O Can I continue to use this drug even after the trial?
O What are my chances of receiving the drug and not a placebo?
O Will I be able to have access to the drug if I receive the placebo during the trial?

The Hepatitis B Foundation newsletter and website www.hepb.org often carries a listing of trials that are looking for volunteers as well as a regularly updated Drug Watch. Also, you may find small ads in your local newspapers. You can also call the Liver Study Unit or GI department of your local research hospital to ask if any trials are starting up in the near future.

CenterWatch is an industry-sponsored listing of clinical trials that are actively recruiting participants. They also offer an e-mail notification service if a trial opens for a possible treatment of HBV. You can go to www.centerwatch.com/patient/trials.html to find more information. The federal government is also a good source of information on clinical trials. You can peruse their comprehensive database at www.clinicaltrials.gov.

Another site, www.thehealthexchange.org, offers a personalized, confidential homepage that keeps track of clinical trials. After you've completed a short trial matching questionnaire and registered with the site, you will be notified when a trial matches your needs.

IN A SENTENCE:

> *In order to avoid unpleasant surprises, you need to know about insurance plans and how to receive maximum coverage.*

HALF-YEAR MILESTONE

Now that you're halfway through your first year with HBV, you've significantly expanded your understanding of HBV and how it affects you and your family, and have:

- ○ LEARNED ABOUT HOW THE VACCINE CAN HELP YOU, YOUR FRIENDS, AND FAMILY.

- ○ DISCOVERED THAT MANY OF THE FEELINGS YOU NOW HAVE ARE SHARED BY OTHERS.

- ○ UNDERSTOOD THAT DEPRESSION IS A COMMON SYMPTOM OF LIVER DISEASE.

- ○ FOUND WAYS TO HELP AND TREAT CHILDREN WITH HBV.

- ○ INFORMED YOURSELF ABOUT WORK ISSUES, INSURANCE, AND CLINICAL TRIALS.

As you now enter the last half of the year, you can expect to further expand your mastery of life with HBV by:

- ○ LEARNING ABOUT TREATMENTS IN DEVELOPMENT.

- ○ FINDING OUT WHO NEEDS TRANSPLANTS AND HOW THEY GET THEM.

- ○ BEING INFORMED ABOUT DRUG INTERACTIONS AND ADDICTION.

- ○ CHANGING YOUR DIET AND ADDING HEALTHY, LOW-FAT FOODS AND FLUIDS.

Treatments in Development

THE FOLLOWING drugs are currently in Phase III trials, and will most likely be on the market soon. These drugs have different strategies and approaches for treating HBV, and are grouped below according to their treatment mechanism.

Nucleoside analogues

As mentioned before, nucleoside analogues interfere with the enzymes that viral DNA needs to replicate. The nucleoside analogue drugs that are most likely to become available on the market are Entecavir, Lobucavir, and **FTC** (**Covaricil**). Studies of these agents are currently taking place, and it is likely that an innovative combination of these new medications has the potential to inhibit HBV replication without mutations so characteristic of Lamivudine. In fact, a cocktail drug very similar to those currently used against HIV therapy will be the rule soon.

Famciclovir belongs to a family of drugs called deoxyguanosine analogues, and has been used successfully against herpes. It has also shown activity against HBV. Larger trials have not delivered its promise of achieving a sustained suppression of HBV DNA or HbeAg seroconversion when used as monotherapy. However its value may lie in using it in combination with

Lamivudine to prevent mutations and this combination has had some promising results. Overall, Famciclovir will most likely not be the drug of choice for treating HBV.

Entecavir. Bristol-Myers Squibb (www.bms.com) is currently testing Entecavir. Like Adefovir and Lamivudine, Entecavir facilitates a reduction of HBV DNA levels, but has a slower rebound after stopping therapy than Lamivudine. It, too, is effective against Lamivudine resistant HBV mutants. Entecavir will most likely be studied in longer-term dosing trials to evaluate its effect on viral replication and cccDNA. Reports from early studies have been quite promising and large-scale clinical trials are being carried out.

There are no long-term studies available about Entecavir, so little is known about your options if you don't seroconvert during therapy or potential side effects. And, since it does have an effect on normal cells, it does carry the risk that it might affect vital cell functions.

Nucleotide Analogues

Adefovir dipivoxil, unlike Lamivudine and others, is a nucleotide analogue inhibitor and was originally formulated to fight the HIV virus. Although it, too, is an HIV hand-me-down, it looks to be very promising for HBV.

Adefovir has had a difficult birth, however: in early clinical trials for HBV some people developed severe kidney problems. The drug has, as a result, undergone new clinical trials with lower dosages and the current tests are evaluating 10 mg and 30 mg once daily. The 10 mg dose is very likely to be approved by the FDA. Some doctors still remember those disastrous early trials, and may need to be reminded that Adefovir has been tested at significantly smaller doses. Many of us have quietly and patiently waited for years for FDA approval of Adefovir.

Adefovir quickly reduces levels of HBV DNA. Early trials at the new dosages show promising results. Although Adefovir appears not to lower levels of HBV DNA as quickly as Lamivudine, no mutations have developed in the clinical trials for those people who had never received prior treatment for their HBV. The drug also appears to be effective for those with precore mutant HBV (a strain of HBV that evolves without the assistance of HBeAg). What is more, liver histology (the amount of inflammation and scarring in your liver) was improved over 48 weeks in 53 percent of people participating in one of the studies.

Adefovir has also been tested for those who are co-infected with HIV, and the results show that it is very effective for those who have developed a resistance to Lamivudine. This is great news, especially given the fact that approximately 10 percent of HIV-infected people are also HBV carriers.

Gilead Sciences, Inc. (www.gilead.com), maker of Adefovir, expects to file for FDA approval in the first half of 2002.

Tenofovir is a nucleotide reverse transcriptase inhibitor. In case you're wondering, a nucleotide is a nucleoside combined with a phosphate (salt of phosphoric acid). Tenofovir is made by Gilead and is marketed for HIV in the United States and Europe as Viread. Tenofovir, like Adefovir, may be another HIV hand-me-down. Tenofovir may be less toxic to kidneys, and may also be effective against mutant HBV. If approved for HBV, it may also be used in combination with other drugs.

Immune system enhancers

In Month 2 we learned about how the HBV vaccine is being used by some people with HBV as treatment for HBV itself. The basic idea is that the vaccine helps our immune system fight the virus and possibly develop antibodies. Unlike nucleoside analogues, which interfere with the virus's ability to reproduce, the following drugs are being developed to super-charge your immune system and help it fight the virus:

Zadaxin (Thymosin 1 alpha). Thymosin 1 alpha, marketed by SciClone (www.sciclone.com) is a synthetic **polypeptide** that has its origin in the thymus gland and is known to have **immunomodulatory** properties (something that suppresses or strengthens the body's immune system). It has been shown to augment the body's natural defenses, and it stops HBV replication without too many side effects. Large-scale studies have failed to show efficacy in clearing HBeAg in people with chronic HBV infection. Zadaxin has two major drawbacks: it is not yet approved for use in the United States and is quite costly. It has, however, been approved in 13 countries. It has been used in combination with Interferon or Lamivudine.

Theradigm, now in phase two trials, is another kind of vaccine therapy that enhances helper T-cell activity, is being developed by Epimmune. Theradigm-HBV has been shown to induce flare in ALT similar to those seen in people taking Interferon. This is significant because those who see a flare in ALT are very often those who go on to seroconvert or even lose the virus completely.

Emerging therapeutic approaches

Nonnucleoside antivirals

Imino Sugars. Two new anti-HBV agents called Imino sugars, also known by the mouthful scientific name N-nonyl-deoxynojirimycin (N-nonyl-DNJ) and N-nonyl-deoxygalactojirimycin (N-nonyl-DGJ), have been shown in early trials to suppress HBV replication. While its antiviral activity may be less aggressive than with Lamivudine, it is comparable to other nucleoside analogues. It is quite possible that Imino sugars will be used in combination with other drugs to fight chronic HBV. And somehow having sugar in the name makes them sound more pleasant and promising.

Deciding which drugs to combine and how to combine them will necessitate long-term study of drug potency, how and where the drugs are activated in our bodies, their effect on cccDNA, and the viral mutations that may develop after long-term use.

GENE AND STEM-CELL THERAPIES

Experiments with gene and stem-cell therapies show great potential. Until recently **gene therapy** still sounded like something out of a science fiction movie. However, the study of transferring genetic material to our cells has the potential to revolutionize medicine much in the way the development of antibiotics and vaccines did in the second half of the last century. The first clinical test of gene therapy was carried out in 1989.

The liver is an important area of study for gene therapy, and not just because hepatitis afflicts so many people around the globe. Many inherited disorders, such as cystic fibrosis, Wilson's disease, hemophilia, and hemocromatosis, also originate in the hepatocytes of the liver.

One strategy for gene therapy would be to use a section of your own liver to cultivate liver cells and then reintroduce them into your body. Yet another would be to remove a significant part of your liver while infusing you with genes. These strategies are radically different in scope to what has been traditionally used against HBV, and it is worth staying informed about them.

The kind of gene therapy envisioned for HBV is called antisense therapy. It would probably make sense to most of us to insert a "good" gene into our bodies to replace the "bad" ones that have been damaged by HBV. But antisense goes against this notion by inserting genes that match the DNA/RNA of the virus in order to inactivate it. It does so by sticking to the virus like Velcro, making it hard for the virus to go out and destroy healthy liver cells.

Preliminary investigations regarding the use of stem cells for treating hepatitis B have been promising. There are a few strategies currently being investigated. One of the more successful aims to isolate bone marrow-derived stem cells (which are progenitors of liver cells) and insert them back into the liver.

IN A SENTENCE:

> *There are many new and promising treatments on the horizon, and it is a good idea to stay informed about them.*

learning

Co-Infection

JUGGLING HBV and other diseases means even more variables and considerations. It also means that your learning curve is even steeper. If, along with HBV, you are found to simultaneously have HIV, HCV, or HDV, then you have what is called a co-infection. If you already have HBV but go on to develop a flare due to Delta (HDV), hepatitis A, or hepatitis E it is then called a superinfection. Delta virus is the most common HBV superinfection.

Having both HBV and HCV adds a twist

If you are co-infected with both HCV and HBV, HCV may call the shots. Three to eighteen percent of those with HBV are co-infected with HCV. Some studies have shown that HCV can actually suppress or eliminate HBV replication. In most people one infection predominates while the other is, for all intents and purposes, dormant. Thus in cases where HBV is the dominant virus, HBV is detectable and HCV isn't, and vice versa. Occasionally both diseases may be active. If this is the case, there is an elevated risk for developing cirrhosis and HCC (liver cancer) compared to infection by either virus on its own.

Having both HBV and HDV is cause for concern

Having both HBV and HDV, however, is like having a supercharger on your Honda. It looks the same, but it goes faster. The hepatitis D virus piggybacks on HBV—in fact, it needs HBV to survive and replicate. It also increases your chances of having fulminant hepatitis. Some of us get HDV and HBV at the same time (co-infection). Others are unlucky enough to get HDV superinfection. This may produce a flare that may last 2–3 weeks, after which the liver enzymes return to their starting point.

Three quarters of those who have both hepatitis B and D go on to develop cirrhosis, and some may even start developing fibrosis or cirrhosis within a few years of infection. For this reason, if you haven't been tested for HDV yet, ask your doctor to include it in your next blood draw.

HBV And HIV

Some studies have found that up to 90 percent of those who are infected with HIV also have or have had HBV. This is, in part, due to the fact that both transmission modes and **epidemiology** (the way a disease behaves) are also very similar. However, only about 10 percent of HIV-positive people become chronic HBV carriers.

HIV unwittingly promotes HBV replication, and when both are present liver disease is more common and tends to progress more rapidly. For this reason having both HBV and HIV can increase your chances of experiencing more liver scarring. And the HIV drug cocktails can be hard on a damaged liver. It's a good idea to be regularly tested for HIV, particularly if you are sexually active.

Be on the watch for liver cancer

Unfortunately, if you're co-infected your chances of having liver cancer are also much greater. It's wise to choose a more aggressive treatment of the predominant virus. The good news here is that the annual incidence of HCC is only 0.1 percent in those who have HBV but are asymptomatic. This annual percentage rises to 1.0 percent in those who are chronic, and 3–10 percent in those with cirrhosis. HCV co-infection makes these percentages rise much higher.

If you're co-infected, it is even more important for you to have blood tests performed 3 to 4 times per year, and you should have an ultrasound once or twice annually. Call your doctor if you experience unusual abdominal pain in your right upper quadrant, swelling in your abdomen, if you bleed or bruise easily, or you experience jaundice.

IN A SENTENCE:

> *Co-infection with other viruses may alter the course of your HBV, so it is essential to be on your guard and undergo regular testing.*

Complications

THANKS TO your new diet, your exercise program, and the medication you may be taking, there's a good chance you won't develop complications due to HBV. Treatments on the horizon will further decrease these chances. However, if you have had HBV since birth or since you were much younger, and you haven't been able to take advantage of medication to fight HBV, there is an increased risk that you may experience some of the complications listed in this chapter.

Hepatitis B can lead to cirrhosis

When your liver cells are damaged and replaced at frequent intervals over the years, your liver can become tough and full of fibrous tissues. When this fibrous tissue spreads to all areas of your liver and starts disfiguring its shape and appearance, this is called cirrhosis. If you are cirrhotic, your doctor may even be able to feel its bumpy surface by pressing down under your rib cage or hear it by tapping on your liver. It is thought that cirrhosis, unlike fibrosis, is not reversible. Once your liver has reached this state, it no longer has the ability to regenerate tissue like it once did.

The presence of cirrhosis may produce the following effects:

○ Less protein is manufactured.
○ Less protein (specifically albumin) means fluid retention (edema).

- ⭕ Less clotting proteins means more bruises and/or bleeding.
- ⭕ More bile pigments in the blood may lead to jaundice.
- ⭕ Bile deposits in the skin can cause intense itching.
- ⭕ Toxins in the brain can cause brain fog, forgetfulness, and encephalopathy.
- ⭕ Drugs cannot be processed as they once were, causing a buildup.
- ⭕ There is increased sensitivity to drugs.
- ⭕ Pressure can build up in the portal vein, causing portal hypertension, which blocks blood flow inside the liver as well as causing the spleen to enlarge. Blood is forced to find another way around the liver and tries to create a new path through new vessels. These vessels can become overloaded and engorged, becoming varices (similar to varicose veins). They are most often found in the stomach and esophagus. They can rupture, causing serious and life-threatening bleeding. This bleeding results in vomiting or excreting blood in stools.
- ⭕ Kidney functions may fail in the presence of advanced cirrhosis, making it difficult or even impossible to remove urine. This may necessitate the use of special medicines or even dialysis.

Although alcohol is one of the common causes of cirrhosis, those with HBV can develop cirrhosis with no warning signs. In fact, it may not even be discovered until the appearance of some of the above-mentioned symptoms.

Cirrhosis can lead to fluid buildup in your abdomen or legs

Ascites are pockets of fluid or large amounts of freely flowing fluids that build up in your abdominal cavity and are usually due to portal hypertension and cirrhosis. They are usually a harbinger of decompensation, and develop within ten years in about half of those with compensated cirrhosis. Untreated, only one third of those who develop ascites survive more than one year without a new liver. Since symptoms include abdominal distention (a pot belly), ascites can be confused with obesity or even pregnancy. Your doctor may decide to test you via ultrasound and aspirating fluid from your abdomen with a needle (paracentesis) to confirm your diagnosis, and various tests may be performed on this fluid to determine the exact cause of the ascites.

There are a few ways your doctor can help control your ascites: bed rest, severe sodium restriction, use of diuretics like Lasix and Aldactone, and manually removing large quantities of fluid by draining the abdomen. Most people with ascites benefit from a combination of these therapies. If the ascites can't be controlled in this manner, you may have a shunt (surgically implanted tube) placed in your abdomen to remove this fluid directly and continuously into a large vein. However, the success rate is low and it is usually associated with complications such as blockages or infection. Another form of shunt is called a TIPS (Transjugular Intrahepatic Portal-Systemic Shunt), which is a tube placed inside your liver to bypass the blood and relieve the portal hypertension. It does not require surgery. It is important to monitor your ascites carefully by weighing yourself daily, noting any sudden changes. One potential life-threatening complication of ascites is spontaneous bacterial peritonitis, in which the fluid becomes infected. This may trigger an episode of bleeding or encephalopathy.

Cirrhosis can lead to hormonal imbalances or changes in your heart or lungs

Hormonal changes due to cirrhosis cause men to literally become more feminine and women to become more masculine. Men may develop enlarged breasts (**gynecomastia**) and testicular atrophy, which leads to reduced sex drive, impotence, and/or sterility.

Liver failure in cirrhosis causes faster circulation of blood and thus a greater burden on your heart and/or lungs. This may cause more fatigue, shortness of breath, and blue discoloration of lips (**cyanosis**).

Flares can happen at any time for many reasons

Acute exacerbation of HBV may occur due to another virus infection (superinfection), HBV activation or following Interferon therapy. Some flares occur as a precursor to good news, in that they sometimes happen just before seroconversion. Flares can also happen if you start drinking again or take hepatotoxic medications or herbs.

Cirrhosis can make you more vulnerable to bruising and bleeding

We need certain proteins for our blood to clot. When the liver is damaged, a lack of these proteins means we bruise or bleed more easily. This also means that it may take longer for your blood to clot after you've been cut or wounded. You may find that you bruise more often or more heavily, or that your skin bleeds more readily if you scratch an area repeatedly.

Cirrhosis can make you more sensitive to medications

When our livers are unable to adequately filter drugs from the blood, these medications can carry out their job longer than expected and eventually build up in the body. This means that we are very often more sensitive to and affected by them. It also means that we may experience more side effects than the average person. For this reason, doctors may prescribe lower doses of some medications in the presence of severe liver disease.

Portal hypertension

As mentioned above, portal hypertension results in the enlargement of your spleen, the development of ascites and the formation of varices. Your doctor should be able to detect any of these symptoms during your visit. This can be detected when a doctor examines you. However, you can examine yourself at home for signs of portal hypertension, by looking for new veins that form on the surface of your abdomen.

If you have cirrhosis you may be asked to undergo an endoscopy

You may be asked to undergo an endoscopy if you have varices (enlarged veins) in your esophagus or stomach. If these varices rupture they can cause severe—even life threatening—bleeding. If you are scheduled to have an endoscopy, you should avoid taking aspirin or other anti-inflammatory drugs. During the procedure, a miniature fiber-optic camera is inserted into your mouth and down into your esophagus and stomach. You will be awake and slightly sedated. The endoscopy allows your doctor to see firsthand how much damage is occurring inside your body.

Encephalopathy

Liver failure can induce mild encephalopathy, or swelling of the brain. Brain fog or changes in behavior may be early signs of encephalopathy. When left untreated, it can cause unconsciousness and even coma. A chest or urinary infection, bacterial peritonitis, changes in the electrolytes in the body, or silent bleeding in the stomach can sometimes precipitate encephalopathy. If you have cirrhosis, inform your family, friends and coworkers about the possibility of these mental and/or behavioral changes, watch out for subtle changes in demeanor or consciousness, and look for any of the above-mentioned complications. These symptoms can be corrected, leading to a disappearance of encephalopathy.

Kidney failure

Functional kidney failure, also known as hepato-renal syndrome, is a dreaded and often fatal complication of advanced cirrhosis. It usually occurs due to circulatory changes taking place because of cirrhosis and portal hypertension, and there is no primary kidney damage. It results in rapid decrease in urine formation and requires early detection and specialized treatment in a hospital. Treatment may include dialysis.

Acute HBV can be deadly

Although cases are quite rare (less than 1 percent), HBV can sometimes strike like lightning, endangering the life of the infected person. When this occurs we call it fulminant HBV. After the normal initial incubation period of about 75 days with or without classic symptoms, some people experience a very rapid escalation of HBV DNA levels in their blood that leads to severe inflammation of the liver. Since this rapid process can lead to encephalopathy and coma, quick identification of the cause is critical.

Fortunately, for those who experience fulminant hepatitis B, a rapid decrease over the following three to six weeks is customary, and very often these people go on to lose the e antigen and develop antibodies. Patients may spontaneously recover. If this happens, no treatment is required. Proper diet and hydration are essential. However, if recovery is not evident, the only option for survival is a liver transplant.

IN A SENTENCE:

> *If you have HBV for many years without realizing it and treating it, or if you have fulminant hepatitis, serious complications may arise; since severe cirrhosis may cause these complications to appear all at once, you must be ultravigilant about any physical, mental, or behavioral changes.*

learning

Transplants

Chances are good that you won't need a new liver

IF YOU recently contracted HBV and were recently diagnosed, chances are quite good that you will never need a new liver, at least not because of your HBV. You will be able to take advantage of Interferon and/or Lamivudine to keep your viral load in check and lower your enzymes, and new medications will be arriving on the market to further protect the health of your liver. However, those who have unknowingly carried the virus for decades and have severe cirrhosis may someday need a liver. It has been determined that without treatment, the average person moves from stage to stage in about 5 years, depending on specific circumstances. That means that from infection, it could take 15–20 years to reach cirrhosis if you aren't taking any medication for HBV. Whatever your stage, you can help reduce your chances of needing a liver by avoiding drugs and alcohol, exercising, avoiding stress, and getting tested regularly.

This chapter provides information about what you need to do in a worst-case scenario.

How do I get on a list?

If you have cirrhosis and your symptoms are getting worse, your hepatologist may tell you to start thinking about a transplant. Your first step will be to contact a hospital that specializes (if your hepatologist's doesn't) in liver transplants. There are over 200 transplant hospitals in the United States. Make an appointment to have tests run to see if you qualify for and are a good candidate for a liver transplant. Your life depends on this decision, so ask plenty of questions. If the hospital gives you a green light, you will be added to the nationwide list.

If you don't mind the possibility of undergoing another complete medical evaluation, you can even consider listing yourself with more than one transplant hospital. That way, if donor organs become available in one area rather than the other, you may have a better chance of getting a liver. This doesn't automatically mean that an organ will become available faster, and each hospital has its own rules about multiple listings. Ask your transplant hospital about their rules. And while you're at it, research the success rates for all of the hospitals you are considering. Teresa did her homework and it paid off: "Our saving grace was the Mayo Clinic in Jacksonville. When all other transplant facilities had a three to four year waiting list, the Mayo's average was only four months because they were newer and wanted to establish their good statistics and prove their efficiency. The other facilities would not do transplants on weekends and were sitting on their laurels. Ralph got a transplant in two months and just in time. And now he's almost back to normal!"

When do I qualify to be put on a list?

Starting in 2002, more objective medical criteria will now be used to rank patients waiting for donated livers, under a new system that was recently approved by the nation's transplant network. This new system, called MELD (Model for End-stage Liver Disease), replaces one that weighed other factors such as the length a patient had been on a waiting list, though people still need to have a minimum listing criteria based on the previous system, known as the "Child-Pugh Classification of severity of liver disease." Although it may help avoid a system in which some doctors encourage patients to get on the list prematurely in the hopes of saving a place in line, it does not erase geographic boundaries that sometimes allow shorter waits in some areas. Status 1 patients—those who become suddenly ill and are not expected to survive more than a week—still will get first dibs on donated livers.

In the new system, everyone will be assigned a number based on the following:

1. Your body's ability to clot blood (prothrombin time)
2. Your ability to break down hemoglobin (bilirubin level)
3. Your kidney function (**creatinine** level)
4. Cause of your liver disease (**cholestatic liver diseases** such as primary biliary cirrhosis (PBC) and primary sclerosing cholangitis (PSC), alcohol-related or otherwise, and HBV)

The higher your score, the better your chance of moving to the head of the list. Those with type O blood or those with type B who have a score above 20 can get O livers. Should a tie occur it would be broken by factoring in total waiting time.

Other considerations may include: the availability of a support system after your transplant, your mental and/or emotional stability, and the availability of health insurance or hard cash (a transplant can cost $300,000–$500,000).

It is hoped that this new system will reduce the number of people who die waiting for a liver. On average, 18,500 people are on the transplant list at any given time. Roughly 10 percent of those on the list die each year before receiving a liver.

Living donation is on the rise

You've undoubtedly heard stories about people who donate one of their kidneys to save someone's life. But have you ever heard about someone donating a part of his or her liver? Living liver donation is on the rise and getting a lot of attention. In fact, living liver donation is the second most common form of organ donation in the United States. In 1989 the first living liver donation took place, and today about 100 are performed annually. Despite this rapid increase, living liver donations represent only 1 percent of the total annual liver transplants. Currently, the majority of living-donor transplants are to children and teens. Friends or family members can donate up to 70 percent of their livers, and within weeks their own livers will completely regenerate. Ask your transplant center about their policies regarding live donation.

Of course, living donation is not without risk. A recent survey reported that four out of 1,000 recent adult transplants worldwide resulted in donor fatalities.

Can I donate organs?

Yes, in some instances. Contrary to popular belief, you can even donate your liver or other organs to another person with HBV or someone who has HBV antibodies, particularly if you have recovered from hepatitis B and don't have any liver damage. It makes sense to do for others what someone might do for you if and when you need a liver, and chances are good that your organ would go to someone who is experiencing the same things you are now. However, whether your organs will be accepted for donation will be decided on a case-by-case basis. It doesn't hurt to sign your driver's license, carry a donor card in your purse or wallet, and tell your family about your wishes to donate an organ.

Success rates for liver transplants are very high

Mercifully, liver transplant survival rates are quite high. About 80–90 percent survive the first year, while roughly 70 percent survive three years. Others stay healthy for many years.

After your transplant you will most likely be able to return to work and enjoy life with even more energy than before. You will, however, have to follow a rigorous program of the following:

○ Daily antirejection medication
○ Regular testing
○ Healthy diet
○ A rehabilitation program to get your body back in shape

Chances are low that you will reinfect your new liver with HBV

Until recently, liver transplants were often denied to those with HBV due to concerns about reinfection of the new liver that could result in premature organ failure. You will be given high doses of intravenous hepatitis B immune globulin (HBIG) to counteract the virus and prevent reinfection of your new liver. Lamivudine, however, may also effectively prevent viral reinfection after liver transplantation, and other drugs in development will also prevent reinfection. Some transplant centers are also using combination of HBIG and Lamivudine to prevent reinfection of the new liver.

Co-infection with HIV may make it harder to get a liver

In the past it was more difficult to qualify for a liver transplant if you had HIV in addition to HBV. In 2001, however, a state medical appeals board in Massachusetts ruled that an HIV patient with liver disease should receive coverage for a liver transplant—coverage that another patient was denied in similar circumstances the previous summer. In these latest hearings it was revealed that since 1997, 14 liver transplants done in Miami and Pittsburgh on HIV patients with severe liver damage were successful, and none experienced a deterioration of their HIV status. This debate will likely continue for many years, since each case will have to be evaluated separately.

Resources

The United Network for Organ Sharing (UNOS) is a private, non-governmental, and nonprofit organization. It provides support to patients, transplant recipients, medical professionals, friends and families, donors, volunteers, and members of the general public who support donation and transplantation. The network works with every transplant hospital, organ procurement organization, and transplant compatibility lab in the United States. You can contact UNOS by dialing (804) 330-8500 and asking for Patient Services. Or call their toll-free number (888) TX INFO-1 or (888) 894-6361 for a liver information kit.

The Children's Liver Association for Support Services (CLASS) is an all-volunteer, nonprofit organization dedicated to serving the emotional, educational, and financial needs of families coping with childhood liver disease and transplantation. Their goal is to be both a service to families and a valuable resource for the medical community.

Transplant Recipients International Organization, Inc. (TRIO) is a non-profit international organization committed to improving the quality of lives touched by the miracle transplantation through support, advocacy, education, and awareness. Through the TRIO International Office in Washington, DC, a network of chapters throughout the United States and the world, TRIO provides a range of services to its community, including awareness, support, education, and advocacy.

Living Donors Online is an online community for living organ donors, potential donors, their families, and medical professionals.

The Coalition on Donation is a not-for-profit alliance of national organizations and local coalitions across the United States that have joined forces to educate the public about organ and tissue donation, correcting misconceptions about donation and creating a greater willingness to donate. Their excellent site even offers e-postcards about donation that you can e-mail to friends, promotional T-shirts, hats, bumper stickers, and sample letters you can adapt and send to your local paper.

United Network for Organ Sharing (UNOS)
1100 Boulders Parkway, Suite 500
P.O. Box 13770
Richmond, VA 23225-8770
www.unos.org

Children's Liver Alliance
3835 Richmond Avenue, Box 190
Staten Island, NY 10312 USA
718-987-6200
www.livertx.org/

Living Donors Online and
International Association of Living Organ Donors, Inc.
705 Cheswich Overlook
Marietta, GA 30067
www.livingdonorsonline.org/index.htm

The Coalition on Donation
Coalition on Donation
1100 Boulders Parkway, Suite 700
Richmond, VA 23225-8770
e-mail: coalition@shareyourlife.org
(804) 330-8620
www.shareyourlife.org

U.S Department of Health and Human Services
Division of Transplantation
5600 Fishers Lane
Room 481
Rockville, MD 20857
(301) 443-7577
www.organdonor.gov

IN A SENTENCE:

Chances are good that you won't need a new liver, but if you do, your chances of survival are very good.

MONTH **9**

living

Addictions

Get help for your addiction

GETTING A diagnosis of HBV when you have an addiction can either jolt you into stopping cold turkey or push you to abuse more aggressively. I hope you will choose to make the choice for positive change in your life. If and when you are ready to get help for your addiction, you have quite a few choices to make. If you feel like you can handle stopping on your own, you can get extra support from groups like Alcoholics Anonymous (AA) or Narcotics Anonymous (NA).

If you feel like you need to reach out for more assistance, you may decide to take advantage of inpatient counseling if you feel like outpatient visits aren't going to keep you from abusing. If you're not sure if you really do have a problem, go to the Alcoholics Anonymous site (www.alcoholics-anonymous.org/) and take their "Is AA for you?" test. It only takes a few minutes, but will give you an objective view about whether treatment is right for you. "If the 12-step approach works for you—great. If it seems offensive, repressive, or irrelevant, use the parts that do work for you," says Pam Ladds, who has considerable experience in working with addiction, "accepting help, being responsible for yourself, and being open to learning are what counts."

Ask yourself a few questions

Do you feel the need to **C**ut down on drinking?
Are you **A**nnoyed by criticism of your drinking?
Do you feel **G**uilty about your drinking?
Do you have a drink upon waking, called an "**E**ye-opener?"

Most alcoholics will answer yes to at least two of these questions. They are called CAGE questions because of the capital letters in key words shown above. But remember, the bottom line of too much alcohol combined with HBV isn't about if you get drunk or not in front of your friends, or if they criticize you; rather, it's simply about the quantity of alcohol you put through your liver every day. We all know people who have an exceedingly high tolerance and who can drink everyone else under the table. That seems fine for them, but no one can know just how much damage is happening in their liver.

Alcohol has two ways of harming your liver: directly and indirectly

It has been proven that not only is alcohol toxic to your liver in a direct way, but that it is immune-mediated, meaning that it actually acts against your immune system, giving HBV a hand. Think of that big rolling boulder that threatens Indiana Jones. You set that ball in motion and help it gain momentum by frequent alcohol intake, but once the ball gains speed it's unstoppable and will eventually run you over, even if you abstain completely. Think twice about pouring yourself another drink.

Find the cause of your addiction and face up to it

Sometimes the road to recovery means facing up to your deepest fears. "I know that my contracting HBV was directly and indirectly related to my use of mood- and mind-altering substances," says Larry, who has been sober for 13 years and narrowly escaped liver failure due to his addictions. "I was not a falling-down kind of drunk either," he adds, "Too many people carry on with HBV and/or HIV as if they weren't a problem. Typically people get clean and sober and then relapse because they can't see the cause of their need to escape from reality. Recovery takes time—time to become aware of your interdependencies. I used to be on the prowl for pleasure and excitement, but now I search for peace and joy."

Treatment can be prohibitively expensive, but there are public programs

You may be disappointed if you think that your insurance will pick up the tab for a 28-day program in the woods in Minnesota. A month in a clinic costs about as much as a new car, and not surprisingly the clinics want the cash up front before you walk in the door. There are however, many local programs that provide free services or sliding scale fees.

Tobacco use may increase your chances of getting liver cancer

Nicotine should become part of your HBV phase-out. When you're smoking you also tend to accompany cigarettes with food and drink, usually caffeinated or full of saturated fats. Some alternate drags on a cigarette with soft drinks, coffee, or alcohol, others with chocolate or candy. This is a real one-two punch on your liver.

Try applying the phase out schedule from Day 2 to your consumption of cigarettes. Nicotine can trick your brain into thinking that you can't ever be happy again if you don't have a cigarette. Nicotine is incredibly insidious and controlling—when I worked at a drug rehab center people who had kicked their heroin habit would puff away in the courtyard of the center even on the coldest Chicago winter days, lamenting the fact that they were still powerless against nicotine.

Set down a few preliminary ground rules to help you get into the quitting mode:

○ Don't smoke in the morning
○ Don't smoke inside a building
○ Don't carry cigarettes with you
○ Take slow, deep breaths when you feel the urge
○ Carry pretzels, rice cakes, baked chips, or lollipops with you
○ Avoid people who smoke and smoke-filled bars and restaurants

The bottom line here is that cigarette smoking may harm your liver and can impede treatment by weighing your system down with a myriad of toxins that remain in your system longer because your liver can't process them fast enough. And studies show that your chances of getting liver cancer increase by at least 1–3% if you smoke.

Using recreational drugs
is like playing Russian roulette

The reason for this is two-fold: how the drugs affect your liver, and how the drugs affect you and your interaction with when you're high. You're much more likely to engage in unsafe sex or high-risk activities like snorting with a shared straw or sharing a needle with someone. You risk both becoming co-infected with HIV, HCV, or other infectious diseases, and you risk infecting others with your HBV.

In addition, you usually have no idea where the drugs you're using come from, the amount of active ingredients in the substance you buy, and what additives they might contain. Some drugs are cut with solvents, cocaine, or over-the-counter medications. Some mushrooms can be hepatotoxic, and Ecstasy can cause you to be severely dehydrated. These drugs will not be processed as quickly when you have liver damage. That means that a bad trip will be a much longer bad trip and it will take much more time for your body to recover.

Some say that of all recreational drugs, marijuana is the least toxic to the liver and may help combat loss of appetite when on Interferon. This may or may not be true, but it is likely that it will also increase your appetite for foods full of fat, sugar, and salt. Others with moderate liver damage have reported increased sense of paranoia and a marked decrease in blood pressure after smoking marijuana.

Drinking alcohol
puts you at risk of developing a fatty liver

Fatty liver (steatosis) is usually caused by alcohol, obesity, or both. Some people with diabetes mellitus also suffer from fatty livers. People with fatty livers can develop inflammation (steatohepatitis) and have progression of their liver disease with fibrosis and cirrhosis. Although fatty liver can lead to cirrhosis, diet and exercise may help avoid the progression of the disease. Losing enough weight to reenter your ideal body weight is key, as well as total avoidance of alcohol and drugs.

IN A SENTENCE:

> *Alcohol and drugs are bad enough on a healthy liver, but when you have HBV, you need to stop both immediately and get help if you can't stop on your own.*

learning

Drugs, Medications, and the Liver

Be vigilant when taking drugs and medications

YOUR LIVER biotransforms, or processes, all drugs in your body to some extent, so if you have liver damage your liver has a hard time dealing with these drugs. You may not have a choice about avoiding certain drugs if you have another, HBV-unrelated condition. If this is the case, your doctor will probably monitor your enzyme levels closely to make sure you aren't damaging any more liver cells than you have to. Generally, if your liver functions exceed normal values by more than 300 percent, your doctor will probably ask you to discontinue taking the medication.

It is very important to inform your doctor about any medications or drugs you're taking, whether they be prescriptions, over-the-counter drugs, herbal remedies, homeopathic cures, or recreational drugs.

Too many drugs forces your liver to create toxins

Under normal conditions, an enzyme called cytochrome P450 converts drugs and toxins into harmless substances so they can be eliminated from your body. But when your system gets overloaded by excessive amounts of drugs, alcohol, or other toxins, these enzymes go into reverse gear, creating more toxins rather than eliminating them. The liver has a threshold for what it can process, and gets a bit overwhelmed when its limit is reached. This is the same dynamic previously described about excessive alcohol consumption, in which an overload creates a damaging momentum in which the inflammation and scarring process accelerates.

Sometimes, even a normal dose of a drug can bring about a reaction that may seem like an allergy, even though a normal dose may have been taken. If you experience fatigue, fever, numbness, and/or a rash, call your doctor to see if she thinks you should discontinue taking the medication.

Even over-the-counter drugs can be hepatotoxic

Tylenol®, Aspirin-Free Excedrin®, and other over-the-counter drugs containing acetaminophen are said to be safe within recommended daily dosages, as long as they aren't taken for more than a few days in a row. You shouldn't take more than one extra-strength Tylenol®—500 mg—every six hours or two every 12 hours. It is best to consult with your doctor if you need to take more acetaminophen or other pain medications such as nonsteroidals (NSAIDS—see box) when you have chronic liver disease, especially cirrhosis.

The following is a list of some of the drugs you should be careful with (and sometimes avoid) due to their hepatotoxicity:

Partial list of potential hepatotoxic medications

○ Acetaminophen (Tylenol® and Paracetamol, if more than 2 g per day is taken, or combined with alcohol, or continued use)

○ Antibiotics like erythromycin

○ Anticancer drugs

○ Antidepressants

○ Antiseizure drugs like barbituates, Phenytoin, Valporate

○ Azoles (i.e., Metronidazole, Fluconazole)

○ Benzodiazepines and other sleeping pills

○ Birth control pills

○ NSAIDS (non-steroidal anti-inflammatory drugs like Advil®, Aleve®, Excedrin®, Ibuprofen, Indomethacin, Motrin®, Midol®, Naproxen, Nurofen, Pamprin®, Orudis, Voltaren, etc.)

○ Isoniazids (Laniazid, Nydrazid) and other antitubercular drugs

○ Steroids

○ Tranquilizers

○ Vitamin A overdose

Do your homework

Even if your primary physician gives you the green light on a certain prescription, it doesn't hurt to either run it by your hepatologist, or consult a drug guide or an online drug information site like Medline Plus (http://medlineplus.gov/), which is run by the National Library of Medicine and is the world's largest database of medical literature.

IN A SENTENCE:

You must be ultravigilant and consult with your hepatologist about any over-the-counter or prescription drugs you are taking or planning to take.

Depression

Depression is normal

STEVE BINGHAM perfectly sums it up: "No two ways about it, chronic hepatitis can get you down. Faced with limited treatment options, myriad of side effects, unsympathetic friends and family, imperfect doctors, and mounting bills, our first inclination is to just lock ourselves in a closet and never come out again. But closets can get boring after a while."

As mentioned before, many people with HBV experience chronic depression. There's nothing mystical about it: feeling tired and sluggish all the time gets you down. And feeling like you're watching the world go by may bring about feelings of loneliness and sadness. Our livers can't always keep up and sometimes don't even allow our minds to fully function, so often we can't tell what is emotional or psychological or what is induced physically. It is important for you to remember that depression can often accompany HBV and is even a direct consequence of Interferon treatment. But with effort it can be treated and overcome.

The causes of depression can come from within you (chemical imbalances, physical disorder, or the presence of toxins in your body) or from the outside (loss of job or loved one, financial problems, etc.) or a combination of internal and external factors.

Remember that you have the power to make positive change that will help you get to a better place.

Depression and HBV have similar symptoms

Although many of us learn to adapt to our diagnosis, hepatitis B can test our patience. Roughly half of the subscribers to the HBV-L support group have said they suffer from depression to some degree. As mentioned above, there are many different factors that can lead us to feeling depressed, but often for someone with HBV biological factors may play a more active role. This is important to remember, so that you don't start chipping away at your self-esteem for all the wrong reasons. When depression accompanies another disease like diabetes, heart disease, or hepatitis, it is called co-occurring depression. And, since many of the symptoms of depression are quite similar to those of HBV, it is good to have a careful look at each one and check the box for the symptoms and origins you think are attributable to each. In the following table, put a check in the box or boxes that best represents your situation.

Is it depression or is it HBV?

	HBV	DEPRESSION	NOT APPLICABLE
Fatigue or listlessness			
Lack of concentration			
Sleep disturbances			
Feelings of sadness			
Lack of appetite			
Impotence or lack of interest in sex			
Thoughts about death			
Feelings of guilt or worthlessness			
Antisocial behavior			
Other			

Don't let your doctor get these symptoms mixed up

You may be quite sure that your feelings are due to HBV, but your doctor may not fully understand the extent of your symptoms and may write the term "somatization disorder" or "hypochondriac" on your chart notes. Seeing "hypochondriac" on your chart is the height of irony, especially when you have a disease with many and varied symptoms. Some have reported being upset by the term "patient is preoccupied with HBV" or "patient complains of multiple symptoms." Don't fret too much about this clinical language, since some of it is medical shop talk that has lost some of its meaning. For example, one of my former doctors wrote the following about me after a visit a few years ago: "patient complains of feeling good."

However, if you feel like your doctor doesn't give enough attention to your feelings and your feelings continue to cause concern, ask the doctor for a referral to a therapist or counselor or ask friends if they have any recommendations. Try to find a therapist who has experience with chronic disease. Not only will they be more understanding of your particular circumstance, but also they will have a better understanding of how to counsel you and treat you if necessary.

Your depression may be seasonal

Seasonal affective disorder (SAD) means that you are affected by changes in seasons. During the fall or winter months, when there is less sunlight, some people develop mild depression. Bright light is thought to counteract SAD by affecting brain chemistry, so therapy involves sitting under special bright lights for at least 30 minutes per day.

Medications may help your depression, but can hurt your liver

There are 2 classes of antidepressants: conventional tricyclic drugs, and the newer selective serotonin reuptake inhibitors (SSRIs, of which Prozac is the first generation), but neither could be classified as liver friendly. If your doctor prescribes antidepressants, you will probably be monitored quite closely for any rise in your liver enzymes. Your doctor may even prescribe a lower dose if you have some liver damage, since these drugs can stay in your system 30 percent longer than in someone with a healthy liver.

Compared to first generation tricyclics, SSRIs had significantly higher rates of diarrhea, nausea, insomnia, and headache. Tricyclic antidepressants had significantly higher rates of dry mouth, constipation, dizziness, blurred vision, and tremors. Less than 1 percent of those who took SSRIs experienced serious adverse effects like bleeding, seizures, or hepatotoxicity.

The bottom line is that it is probably best to consult with your specialist before you use antidepressants if you have liver disease. Ask your doctor about a drug called amitryptyline, which may be good for short-term use.

Some people with depression qualify for disability

According to the National Institute of Mental Health, major depression is the leading cause of disability in the United States and worldwide. It may seem ironic, but even if you have cirrhosis you may not necessarily qualify for disability payments. But some people with HBV have managed to get approved because of documented depression. If you have been suffering from chronic depression along with your HBV, keep notes about your condition and how it affects your work and daily functioning. It may help you qualify for disability much sooner than with HBV alone.

Search the Web for resources and diagnostic tests

The electronic bulletin boards of www.depressionforums.com are informative and well organized. News groups such as alt.support.depression and soc.support.depression.misc can also make you feel like you're not alone. You may have to call your Internet service provider to find out what your news server (NNTP) address is.

The National Depressive and Manic-Depressive Association educates patients, families, professionals, and the public concerning the nature of depressive and manic-depressive illnesses as treatable medical diseases, and fosters self-help for patients and families. They also have a helpful, nationwide support-group database on their website: www.ndmda.org/.

You can take online tests to see if you indeed have depression. Here are just a few of the many sites available online:

New York University School of Medicine:
    www.med.nyu.edu/Psych/screens/depres.html
Depression Screening.org:
    depression-screening.org/screeningtest/screeningtest.htm
Psych Central: psychcentral.com/depquiz.htm

Watch out for bad shamans

What is a bad shaman? A good shaman is someone who helps you heal, while a bad shaman can be a detriment to your treatment regimen. We can unwittingly go for years believing what someone says, without questioning the veracity of his or her opinion. Some start from our earliest years, like a teacher who tells us that we're better at math than art. Others come later, when people project their own ideas onto our personality. Learning to identify situations in which someone puts negative ideas into your head (either intentionally or accidentally) is healthy, since you really do have the power to overcome negative suggestions. Question everything you hear, and don't let bad shamans pull you down. You are in charge of deciding what will make you happy.

Most cases of depression can be successfully treated by stopping Interferon treatment, medication, therapy, diet and exercise, or a combination of some or all of these. Get help.

Resources

National Depressive and Manic-Depressive Association
730 N. Franklin Street, Suite 501
Chicago, IL 60610-7204
(800) 826-3632
www.ndmda.org/

National Foundation for Depressive Illness
P.O. Box 2257
New York, NY 100116.
(800) 239-1295
www.depression.org/

American Psychological Association
750 First Street, NE
Washington, DC 20002-4242
(800) 374-2721
TDD/TTY: 202-336-6123
www.apa.org/

IN A SENTENCE:

> *Depression is a common occurrence in those with HBV and can be effectively managed.*

learning

Common HBV Misconceptions

IF YOU have hepatitis B, it may sometimes seem like yours is the most misunderstood and misinterpreted of the world's most common diseases. This is very likely due to the fact that if we learned anything about HBV in school, from doctors, or from the media over the years, it is usually quite outdated due to very recent research and novel treatments. We can hardly expect everyone to keep up with all of the recent developments—there are dozens of diseases for doctors to juggle—but we must be attentive not to disseminate HBV falsehoods that could affect our livers and our lives. No matter how unfair it may seem given how much we spend for medical treatment, the burden of responsibility for staying informed falls squarely on your shoulders.

For this reason, I have chosen to list the most common misconceptions that people have about HBV, in the hope that you will be forewarned and vigilant about them. These can act as traps that lead you to go untested when you should be tested or untreated when you should be treated.

"There are no available treatments for HBV"

Many of us, especially those diagnosed before the mid-1990s, may be quite convinced that there are no available treatments for

HBV. Kim's experience is, unfortunately, a classic example of how a total lack of information leads to subsequent and unnecessary infection. "When my husband was first diagnosed with HBV, they told him and just sent him on his way. He had no idea what it was or what he was to do. And being who he is, he just said, 'Hmph,' and went about his life. When he met me and I was later diagnosed with it, he realized that it was something serious. And being highly educated, I felt pretty ignorant when I found out I had contracted it."

It's normal to feel rather ignorant when you're diagnosed. To add insult to injury, many of us are told that there isn't anything we can do to fight HBV except abstain from alcohol. A majority of those I interviewed were told at some time over the past few years that there were no treatments for HBV. Fortunately, none of these misinformed medical professionals were hepatologists.

"There's no need to have the vaccine"

There is precious little information circulating about the availability and efficacy of the HBV vaccine, especially for adults. Ironically, most children must receive the vaccine series as part of a school entry requirement, but no one ever checks to see if their parents have HBV or have received the vaccine. Here is Kim again: "I had had both my daughters immunized, the first one at birth, just because it was part of a package of shots recommended. But like a lot of people out there, I never had a doctor suggest I have the 3-shot series. I knew nothing about it." John Clark shares this frustration about a seemingly total lack of HBV-related prevention: "I felt if my doctors did better jobs *preventing* me from disease rather than giving me only 5 minutes or so for light check-ups of what disease I may be having, I might not have HBV today. Many people out there, whom I personally know, still don't know there are vaccines to protect them. I wish we all are better educated about not only HBV, but also *all* transmittable diseases that we can prevent."

Sometimes doctors are so focused on the patient in front of them that they forget to consider the bigger picture. In Teresa's case, her husband had just been diagnosed not just with HBV, but also with end-stage cirrhosis. "I was not offered the hep B vaccine until I switched primary care providers 3 times, and found a very caring compassionate doctor who knew what he was doing." Medical professional don't usually say the vaccine isn't necessary per se. They just don't usually ask if you've ever had the vaccine, even if you are known to be part of a high-risk group. The "HBV vaccine question" should be included in new-patient questionnaires and patient checklists that nurses or doctors use with all of their patients.

However, it is also true that many patients don't feel comfortable discussing their sexual habits or other personal details like drug use or unsafe sexual practices with their physicians. Studies show, for example, that gay and bisexual men whose doctors are aware of their sexual preference have a much better chance of getting needed attention, including important vaccinations.

There is another, more drastic variation of HBV vaccine misinformation, and it is sadly still relatively widespread. Believe it or not, some doctors are still telling patients that there is no vaccine against HBV.

"You had the vaccine so you have nothing to worry about"

Unfortunately, even if you've had a proactive doctor that pops the HBV vaccine question, you may have been injected only with a false sense of security if the doctor never bothered to check you for HBV antigens beforehand. There is a very slight chance that your or your partner's immune system did not develop HBV antibodies even if the full series of three shots was administered. Although it is unlikely and occurrences are quite rare, it is possible to be infected with mutated HBV or be contagious even if you have developed surface antibodies. In most cases, however, your immune system has a built-in memory of the surface antibody and will react to HBV antigens even if no antibodies show in a spot-check of your antibody titres. As a precaution, it is usually wise for your partner and family to check titres every 10 years or so.

"Treatments are available but aren't effective"

Many doctors have quite rightly held that Interferon isn't effective enough (in fact only 20 percent have a positive outcome) and lowered our quality of life too much. However, not all of those taking Interferon experience serious side effects, and Interferon does offer one possibility that nothing else does: a shot at being relatively cured. Other people I've interviewed have had doctors tell them that Lamivudine is not yet FDA approved.

"You're cured"

We've all heard our doctor speak these words in our dreams. Some of us, however, have even heard them from actual doctors. There are numerous misconceptions about what constitutes actually being cured. People who have recently been infected and have suffered from six months or less of acute HBV and gone on to develop HBsAb are, indeed, cured. Yet some medical professionals mistakenly believe that if we lose HBeAg and develop the e antibody we are cured. Developing HBeAb is no doubt a cause for celebration. It is just the first—though major—hurdle. There is debate about whether someone who develops the S-antibody (HBsAb) can rightly be called *cured*, as blood HBV DNA can be present especially in the liver even in the presence of HBsAb. This is known as occult infection. In long-term chronic HBV, the spare parts of HBV virus actually integrate with our own DNA, making it virtually impossible to eradicate since our own bodies produce it.

There are no easy black-and-white truths about HBV, despite the efforts of many to reduce it to such. Even if we develop all of our antibodies, if we have had HBV for many years we still may have to deal with fibrosis and complications, especially if cirrhosis is present. *Cured* can sometimes be a misleading notion and cruel irony if you're left with a ravaged liver, ascites, and varices.

"You have no symptoms so you don't need to be treated"

It is important to remember that the majority of people with HBV have no symptoms whatsoever. It's HBV's Trojan horse strategy for spreading the virus: a false façade of health with a dangerous passenger inside. HBV likes to keep us feeling well but infectious so long that often decades pass before we feel the first symptoms.

It's quite common for doctors to shy away from treating if they haven't had too much experience with HBV. If I had listened to my primary physician, for example, I may have developed cirrhosis years ago.

"If you stop drinking and smoking you'll get better"

Diabetics commiserate about the run-ins they have with what they call the sugar police—those people who feel the need to check up on their eating habits. Those with HBV have their own police, and some of them double-duty as our doctors, family members, and colleagues. This is an inversion of the "just don't drink alcohol" misconception, in that sometimes people who aren't informed about liver disease see the problem from their own limited perspective.

Those who have never experienced fatigue firsthand can't imagine that our problems stem from something much more complex than what we eat and drink, though our diet, along with avoidance of toxins, is absolutely critical to our well-being. If the worst someone has experienced is a tummy ache or hangover, it seems logical to them that all we have to do is avoid eating or drinking the wrong things. But one of the hardest tests of our spirit and endurance is when HBV marches on even if we've rigorously followed every possible dietary limitation, exercised, and meditated.

There are dozens of other pitfalls

At the top of the classification of HBV misinformation: the belief that herbs like milk thistle don't work or that herbs work much better than traditional Western medicine. Another misconception is that some doctors, having studied about Blumberg's research with the Australian antigen, mistakenly think that HBV occurs only in Australia or Asia, or that it is quite a rare disease. Some may think that anyone with HBV can reap benefit from a shot of immunoglobulin or steroids, or from higher doses of Lamivudine. Another common error is thinking that since HBV is also known as serum hepatitis, you can only get it from infected blood.

There are also bad shamans who would have us believe that we can't have children or ever have sex again. No wonder it is common for those who have been recently diagnosed to have the feeling that there is no hope for them, and that they have no business contemplating a long and happy future ahead of them. I often hear people say that if they had blindly accepted what their doctor told them, they would be sitting at home waiting to die.

For years Ian went to his doctor in Scotland, complaining about fatigue. His doctor said he worked too hard and was just getting older. "He eventually sent me to a psychiatrist, who told me I was an anxious person. Then, my doctor was ill and a temporary doctor had me diagnosed within eight weeks. The new doctor said my liver might have given out within five or ten years without treatment. Where would I be now, fifteen years later, if my first doctor hadn't been sick that day?"

The bottom line: Don't take any information about HBV for granted. Double-check everything you hear from anyone (doctor/nurse/website/friend/support group) with one of your other sources. Compare notes with your support group. Your life is too precious to make blind assumptions about others' blind assumptions.

IN A SENTENCE:

Since there are many misconceptions about HBV, you should be forewarned and vigilant about them.

Fluids

Staying hydrated is important

A RECENT study funded by the bottled water industry found that only one third of Americans drinks the recommended daily amount of water (eight or more glasses per day), and 11 percent of those questioned said they never drink any water at all. Does that sound like you? Some doctors believe that poor hydration is the reason for recent increases in allergies and other seemingly unrelated ailments like headaches.

We tend to stick to our sodas, coffee, tea, and other caffeinated drinks, thinking that we're still putting enough fluids into our bodies. Caffeine, however, acts as a diuretic, causing the body to lose fluid due to increased urination. And many of these drinks contain various artificial colors and preservatives. The summer is a particularly critical time to keep hydrated, as water is essential to every single cellular process in our body. Water, for example, helps the liver remove wastes, control our body temperature, and lubricate joints.

Ironically, some of the early and mild signs of dehydration mirror HBV symptoms: dizziness, headaches, fatigue, lightheadedness, irritability, and dark circles under your eyes. Don't wait until you are thirsty to have a glass of water—thirst is not a very effective gauge of improper hydration. If you feel the need to urinate less than every 4–5 hours, chances are good that you're not getting enough.

A side note: the FDA regulates bottled water, while your tap water is regulated by the Environmental Protection Agency. I have a little more faith in the FDA.

Get in the habit of watering down

We're already getting our taste buds accustomed to less salt, fat, and sugar, so now it is time to start watering everything down. Adding 50 percent filtered water is an excellent method for keeping hydrated and avoiding excess sugar, caffeine, and artificial colors. It also may help us slim down a bit.

It will sound awful at first, but try gradually adding water to your favorite drinks. Orange juice, for example, can be hard to stomach for some people with chronic hepatitis, due to the concentrated sugar and acid. Try adding water the next time you have juice. For a few weeks add 25 percent, and then gradually move up to 50 percent or more. This works well for other juices, coffee/decaf, sodas, and teas. It is certain that after a few months of gradual dilution you will not want to go back to your old ways. You may want to avoid icy drinks as well—many of my interviewees say they have poor tolerance for cold drinks.

Herbal teas can replace soft drinks

The U.S. government does not regulate herbal teas. However, if the **Food and Drug Administration** says a substance is safe for use in foods, you can probably assume that it won't harm you as a tea unless you have a specific allergy. As a general rule, avoid teas or blends that contain unfamiliar ingredients unless you've done some research about them. Rather, look for contents that may normally be part of your diet (such as mint, citrus, berries, or dried fruit); choose them over unfamiliar substances.

If you can't be absolutely sure about what plants are in your yard, don't try to make teas out of them. In my backyard, for example, I have a few dozen herbs growing in a rather tangled mess. The mint, fennel, sage, and rosemary would make a great brew, but the comfrey leaves that are intertwined would be toxic to my liver and could send me to the hospital. Don't take chances unless you feel 100 percent sure about the plant.

Quite a few people have mentioned how beneficial a cup of chamomile is in the evening—it warms you up and calms you down, and helps you get a good night's sleep. I make extra and enjoy it at room temperature in the morning.

Here is a partial list of other teas that help your liver:

○ Burdock
○ Cinnamon
○ Dandelion
○ Fennel
○ Ginger
○ Licorice
○ Milk thistle
○ Peppermint (avoid peppermint tincture, which can be toxic)
○ Roasted chicory (a good coffee substitute)
○ Schizandra

Traditional Medicinals® has been making herbal teas for 25 years and has a wide variety of great handcrafted organic herbal teas, including my favorite, "Everyday Detox." You can even get a free sample and learn more about teas in general by visiting their site: www.traditionalmedicinals.com.

Green tea

Green tea is made from fresh, unfermented tea leaves. The effects of tea have been known since ancient times. Although studies on green tea began in the 1920s, it wasn't until the 1980s that animal experiments investigated its physiological effects. This research showed that green tea contains many beneficial and antioxidant substances as well as vitamins A, C, and E. **Catechin**, an antioxidant found in green tea, has shown to have anticancer and antiviral properties, among others. Free radicals are molecules and pieces of molecules that can damage the body at the cellular level, increasing our risk of cancer, heart disease, and other diseases. Catechins destroy free radicals. Green tea also aids the digestion process and decreases fat content in the blood, and it contains minerals like selenium and manganese, as well as potassium and fluoride. Since we're no longer drinking tap water, green tea can be a good source of fluoride for protecting your teeth and gums.

Decaffeinated green tea may lose its nutritional components if it is put through a water-based decaffeination process. You can perform your own decaffeination process at home by pouring a small amount of boiling water on your green tea leaves then letting it steep for thirty seconds. Pour off this water and make your pot of tea as normal with the leaves that have been pre-steeped.

Try to drink skim milk, no-fat milk, or no milk at all

Skim milk and fat-free milk have the same amount of protein as whole milk. And the protein in milk is a high-quality protein that is useful for your liver. If you have cirrhosis, you may want to avoid concentrated doses of protein, so some people with HBV avoid milk altogether. If you don't drink milk and are concerned about calcium deficiency, you can still get plenty of calcium from spinach, greens (mustard, collard, turnip), broccoli, and cabbage. Arugula, for example, contains five times more calcium than 2 percent milk (per 100 calories).

Enjoy a smoothie

Throw a banana, a handful of ice cubes, and a cup of low or nonfat unflavored yogurt in your blender as a starting point for your smoothy. Then add whatever fresh ingredients you have on hand in your kitchen: berries, peanut butter, juice etc. Kids love experimenting with the blender. Smoothies are a good alternative to a dinner if you get home late and don't want to go to bed on a full stomach.

What to drink at a restaurant

Keep a supply of herbal teas or decaf packets in your pocket or purse. Ask if the tap water is filtered before filling your glass, or order a bottle of fancy mineral water and add lime. You can order decaf along with a large cup of ice and make iced decaf. Or order a nonalcoholic beer or Virgin Mary (with tomato juice, as it has less sodium).

IN A SENTENCE:

> *When you have HBV it is particularly important to stay hydrated with filtered water or fluids that do not contain caffeine or excessive amounts of fat, sugar, preservatives, or artificial colors.*

Phasing In
Liver-Friendly Foods

WE NOW know a little bit about nutrition and we've already started phasing out unhealthy foods. Now it is time to start the phase-in period, where we get creative and find new provisions that will satisfy us just as much or more than the ones we left behind. Getting this to work for you takes a little time and effort, but in time you will adjust your palate and get used to driving out of your way to stock up on harder-to-find healthy foods. In this chapter I will give you a few pointers for pleasing your tastebuds while loving your liver.

Create a new low-fat strategy before you go to the grocery store

Spend a good chunk of your time in the produce department. Before you go shopping, take a new vegetarian recipe along with you. Try to find a recipe that calls for vegetables you're not accustomed to eating. Focusing on gathering ingredients for a new healthy recipe will help you avoid putting all those other processed foods in your basket.

Choose those vegetables that are the most colorful. As a general rule, the more color there is, the more vitamins and minerals there are. Cruciferous vegetables like broccoli, cauliflower, kale, mustard greens, radish, bok choy, and brussel sprouts not only provide nutrients, but they also help detoxify the liver.

Buy whole grain bread and pasta, and try to make at least one bean dish per week. If you can't avoid red meat, choose the leanest cuts available and limit yourself to small portions.

All this may sound like a supreme nuisance, particularly to those who have reduced their culinary skills to dialing the local pizza parlor or pushing the frozen dinner button on their microwaves. Get your friends or partner involved in discovering new low-fat and healthy recipes. Start a weekly low-fat potluck dinner or round-robin lunch club at work. Fellowship and laughter in the kitchen are as therapeutic as any medicine or diet. Watching TV while you're eating is a bad habit and can sometimes be hard to stomach on many levels. It will be hard for your lentil stew to compete with all those mouth-watering burger commercials.

Keep your kitchen stocked with real food

Many find that keeping their kitchen stocked with tasty, low-fat foods helps keep them on track. Stock up on dried fruit, nuts, oatmeal, whole-wheat crackers, hot cereals, granola, whole wheat pasta, brown rice, baked chips, and other goodies. Keep large bags of mixed vegetables in your freezer to make quick vegetarian stir-frys with seitan (wheat-based meat alternative), tempeh (soy cake), or tofu (soy curd). I like to keep cans of turnip or collard greens and kale on hand to mix in soup or season with garlic and onions. Stock up on veggie burgers, salmon burgers, soy or bean burgers, or turkey burgers made without dark meat or skin. Having them at hand will make all the difference. Be on the lookout for the following liver-friendly brands: Eden, Cascadian Farm, Fantastic Foods, Health Valley, Hain, and Moir Glen. They all have tasty prepared foods with low sodium and low fat.

Remember: making your own meals from scratch isn't necessarily just extra work. It's about slowing down, savoring life with loved ones, and taking care of yourself.

What if I can't avoid going to fast food places?

I don't have to tell you that they're ubiquitous—and sometimes unavoidable. If you can't avoid eating at fast food establishments, take time to check the ingredients and make smart choices. Here are a few tips to help you lower your sodium and saturated fat intake:

Choose grilled chicken sandwiches and hold the mayo. The Chicken McGrill, Wendy's Grilled Chicken Sandwich, and the Burger King's BK Broiler all have only 7 grams of fat if you hold the mayo.

Stay away from cheeseburgers. To help you place this into perspective, a Whopper has 47 grams of fat, 17 of which are saturated. The Big & Tasty with Cheese has five times as much fat as the Chicken McGrill, with 37 grams of fat, 12 of which are saturated. The Big & Tasty also has 1210 mg of sodium, about half of your daily intake, and you haven't even counted your fries yet.

Have a salad, hold the dressing. With the exception of taco salads, having a fresh salad is a good bet, as long as your steer clear of blue cheese, French, Caesar, or other creamy dressings. One packet of Wendy's blue cheese salad dressing has more saturated fat than a bacon cheeseburger! Ask for a fat free dressing. When you're in a place that has packets of lemon juice or olive oil and vinegar, swipe as many as you can and keep them in your purse or briefcase.

Low cal drinks. In order to avoid the huge diet drinks, ask for a decaf and a large cup of ice and make your own iced decaf coffee, or put a few fingers of lemonade in your cup, then fill the rest with water.

Breakfast. The breakfast sandwiches have as much saturated fat and sodium as the burgers, so opt for the Fruit and Yogurt Parfait at McDonald's. If you need something hot in your stomach in the morning, gobble up an English muffin with jelly or an Egg McMuffin without meat.

Have a sub. Subway offers a low fat selection of sandwiches called the "7 Under 6™ each offering less than 6 grams of saturated fat.

For more information, you can download nutrition charts from most of the franchises' websites.

A liver-friendly diet doesn't have to be boring. Here are a few ideas for tasty, low-fat meals:

Breakfast	Oatmeal with fresh blueberries
	Whole wheat French toast with applesauce
	Granola with fresh raspberries and fat-free milk
	Low-fat or fat-free yogurt with granola
	Wheat toast and organic peanut butter with banana
Lunch	Chicken or turkey sandwich with arugula and tomato
	Tuna salad sandwich with fat-free or soy mayo
	Cold brown rice salad with tomatoes, boiled eggs, tuna, and olives
	California Rolls (vegetarian sushi) and light miso soup

Dinner	Mesclun salad with walnuts, apples, and dried cranberries; vinaigrette
	Grilled salmon with steamed artichokes
	Health Valley Vegetarian Chili with carrot, orange, and onion salad
	Homemade cabbage soup
	Whole-wheat pasta shells with roasted cherry tomatoes, basil, and black olives
Dessert	Fresh raspberries and low-fat yogurt
	Applesauce
	Baked pears with citrus juice
	Tropical fruit salad
	Fresh blueberries and frozen yogurt

Snacks

Even if we're being careful at meal times, we may be very tempted between meals. To forestall being seduced by the aroma of microwave popcorn in your office or home, stock up on snacks that you can eat with a clean conscience.

Rice cakes. Rice cakes have fueled the writing of this book. Last week there was a sale on rice cakes at the grocery. The cashier must have been a little concerned about me, because I had 25 bags of them in my cart. Only $1.09 each, too! Here's the best part. They have no fat, no cholesterol, and no salt. Most have no sugar, preservatives, or food coloring. The plain variety has only 45 calories per cake and a balanced amount of carbs to give you instant energy without weighing you down. Wait! However, the caramel apple cinnamon and white cheese-flavored rice cakes are just as unhealthy as chocolate chip cookies or potato chips.

Look at the label to make sure that your rice cakes are made with whole grain brown rice and not popped corn. Some of the varieties made with corn can contain a lot of sodium. And if the taste is too dull for your taste buds, you can spread applesauce or peanut butter on top, or you can even lightly rub a clove of garlic on top.

Pretzels. Have a good look at the label on pretzels. Most brands have an excessive amount of salt and hydrogenated oil. But at health food stores or larger supermarkets, you may be able to find unsalted pretzels with oat or whole-wheat flours and no added oil.

Japanese snacks. Dried peas with horseradish powder? Rice crackers with seaweed? Yes! Most of these imports are fat- and cholesterol-free, low in sodium, and contain only rice, soy sauce, red pepper, and water. Can you say that about any American snack? Experiment with different shapes, brands, and varieties, but check to make sure your brand doesn't contain any or too much MSG (monosodium glutamate). Again, it will take a few weeks to become accustomed to the different tastes, but these snacks are very tasty and satisfying.

Single-serving snacks for kids. Put small packages of cereal, raisins, seeds, applesauce, or crackers in your desk or in your car.

Avoid building up resentment

It's hard to watch others enjoy things that you can't eat. But it's good to know that caring for your liver also helps your arteries, skin, kidneys, lungs, and just about every other organ in your body. The key to avoid building up resentment is to make eating healthy foods something you do not because you're forced to, but because you want to treat your body well.

IN A SENTENCE:

> *Altering your diet doesn't have to be hard, as there are many low-fat, healthy foods to choose from.*

MONTH **12**

living

Your Future with HBV

When will I recover from HBV or be cured?

We're close to the end of your first year with HBV, so it might be helpful to review statistics about the probable course of your HBV in the future and the likelihood of a full or partial recovery from it. Remember that out of 100 susceptible adults who come into contact with HBV, 90–95 will develop acute hepatitis B and recover completely. Of the 90–95 who get acute hepatitis B, less than 1 will develop life-threatening fulminant HBV. All of those who are acute will recover (except the unlucky person who experiences fulminant HBV), and most will do so without ever knowing that they've even come into contact with the virus. Fortunately, acute HBV confers lifetime immunity from subsequent HBV infection. However around 5–10 percent of cases do not recover, developing chronic hepatitis. Over the past year we've learned that this is far from a death sentence. Here is a quick rundown of what your chances are of clearing the virus or developing complications:

- ○ Spontaneously clearing the virus = 1 percent per year
- ○ Developing fibrosis and/or cirrhosis = 25 percent
- ○ Developing liver cancer = 5 percent

The progression to **chronicity** (being chronic) depends upon your age at infection (the younger you are, the more likely you will become chronic), and your immune system's ability to fight the virus. Here is a quick overview of your chances of getting help from currently available treatments:

○ Currently available treatments offer a 10 percent chance of a cure
○ Currently available treatments offer a 40 percent chance of stopping viral replication

If you continue to have active virus replication, you are at risk of developing progressive liver disease. As mentioned before, if you develop resistance to an HBV drug you are at risk for ramping up to more inflammation and scarring. However, if you do not have advanced cirrhosis or complications, you will be able to lead a normal life with a modified lifestyle. It is possible you may never get rid of HBV, but you can certainly keep it under control.

You can manage your expectations about what may happen in the future

As mentioned throughout this book, being proactive about both your overall health and your health care is critical. You must take responsibility and also be organized especially regarding health care providers, whose assistance you will depend upon. Be responsible for not taking any information for granted, not even that which your doctor tells you. You can't assume that everyone knows as much as you do about HBV.

If you are infectious, you need to protect your family and loved ones by observing universal precautions. Your proactive efforts to protect your liver will pay off.

Not everyone will develop complications

These days, only one fourth of those with HBV develop complications, and with good care and treatment, even those can be controlled. The key to avoiding complications is early detection. The gold standard of early detection is a liver biopsy, along with ultrasounds, AFP tests, frequent liver panels, and doctors' visits. However, if you can't even remember your last visit to your doctor or hepatologist, you are not promoting early detection.

Here is a pop quiz to see if you are being proactive about early detection:

What is your viral load? _____

How was your last biopsy
   graded? _____

What are your current viral markers? _____

When was your last doctor's visit? (mm/yy) _____

When was your last ultrasound? (mm/yy) _____

If you have a perfect score and your visits were recent, you are doing everything you can to promote early detection. Given that you've had this disease for at least a year now, anything less than a perfect score is, quite frankly, unacceptable. You and your liver deserve better than that.

The survival rate for HBV depends on you

A positive, proactive attitude along with the necessary eagerness to protect your liver will ensure your survival. The natural history of HBV infection with cirrhosis leads to an 85 percent five-year survival rate in those with compensated disease, but only 14 percent in those with decompensated disease. Since you can affect this outcome by exercising, avoiding stress, altering your diet, and keeping informed about HBV and its treatment, you have an edge on survival.

Will I require a transplant and what is its outcome?

If you have a prolonged course of decompensated cirrhosis, you will indeed eventually need a liver transplant. Currently posttransplant survival is roughly 80–90 percent after one year, and approaches 70 percent at the end of three years. Reinfection with HBV can now be prevented in most cases with the use of hepatitis B immunoglobulin and Lamivudine and possibly from newer drugs like Adefovir.

Will I get liver cancer?

The development of cancer is closely related to the severity of the underlying liver disease. The annual incidence of liver cancer is only 0.1 percent in asymptomatic HBsAg individuals, and 1 percent in patients with chronic hepatitis B, but increases to 3–10 percent in patients with cirrhosis.

IN A SENTENCE:

> *It's important to know what your chances are of developing serious liver disease or liver cancer, so that you can be vigilant and put into effect the preventative measures you've learned in this book.*

learning

Taking Stock:
An Inventory
of Personal Growth

"If I look carefully, I live happy with a sad fate."

MICHELANGELO BUONAROTTI

IT'S BEEN a long and difficult year, and you've learned and changed and grown so much this year, that looking back at the past might possibly give you a sense of vertigo. Now's the perfect time to benchmark your progress and gauge both how far along you've come, and where you still want to go both physically and emotionally. Overall, you've probably gained a new perspective on medicine, and what it means to treat yourself. You now know that there are so many factors involved besides just what pills you're popping.

It's also time to start reaping the fruits of your life with HBV. Having this virus is like having a really great teacher. In fact, studies show that people who view their illness as an opportunity for growth have better medical results. You've almost certainly simplified your life, and you have a much better idea of what really matters. You've simplified your tastes and are able to find pleasure in small things.

HBV *helps you get more out of life*

Denny Norton's words are archetypal regarding this positive and subtle shift in perception: "What once seemed so devastating has actually become a 'friend.' This virus has taught me to enjoy what I have and feel grateful. I've learned to make NOW important and satisfying. I no longer worry about the past or the future. I can now take whatever comes and make the best of it. I surely wish I could have learned all of this when I was healthy!" Rodolfo agrees: "I have grown closer to every single member of my immediate family and continue to reach out fearlessly where before there was trepidation. It's strange, but I feel more alive after this diagnosis. I also like myself better."

Here are a few ways that you can objectify your progress:

○ Track your ALT and AST and viral load: Take a moment now and organize your test results if you haven't done it already.
○ Rate your fatigue with a point score in your diary, calendar, or on your computer calendar program.
○ Read over old e-mails from a year ago—sometimes we edit the past and forget how we were really feeling. Fortunately, if you keep old e-mails and actually express your feelings to friends, you probably have a pretty good record of how you were feeling. Go back over them now to see how your perception, energy, and outlook have changed.
○ Get feedback from friends and relatives about how they've seen you change over the past year.
○ Look at pictures: when I see pictures of me during the period I had ALT and AST above 500, I can hardly believe I'm looking at a picture of myself. Seeing those old pictures is the fastest way I know to feel really great about my progress.

Looking at your world, listening to your spirit

What do we mean when we say holistic health and mind, body, and spirit? We're hearing these terms so often these days that they ring in the ear like the tired language of advertising. I'm beginning to think that being holistic is about integrating what we do, see, and believe, in addition to how we think about our disease. It's healthy to expand our definition of healing and our responsibility for it. Our HBV lives are the perfect testing ground for this approach. If we ponder for a moment all the choices that we have to make every day, we have the ability to develop patterns for choosing the paths that will take us to wellness.

Taking the path that takes me away from what others would call "progress" has worked well for me. For example, I avoid TV and don't own a microwave or a dishwasher. I have an unlisted number with caller ID. I try my best to avoid processed foods with ingredients I can't pronounce, and I go out of my way to buy bread from a bakery that doesn't use hydrogenated oil or preservatives. I send away for seeds that haven't been genetically altered. I started developing friendships with people who also take care of their bodies and minds, and have made the difficult decision to avoid negative people. I have made the choice to become invisible to telemarketers, advertisers, researchers, chemical engineers, pessimists, politicians, and the people who build strip-malls. Would I have done all these things had I not been diagnosed?

Balance is key to living with HBV

I've chosen to speak about these things in a learning section to demonstrate how broad the definition of healing can be and how much power we have to effect real change for ourselves. Here's a homegrown wellness manifesto—a few principles we can follow to guide ourselves toward wellness.

Information. Gather medical research and news about alternative medicine. Read labels. Once you've gathered the information, discard most of it and keep the bits that resonate with your body and mind. Gradually weave what you've learned into your daily rituals.

Introspection. Close your eyes every so often and get back in touch with your heart. It's not rocket science. Good thinking doesn't always happen while you're in the supermarket or speeding down the highway. Ask yourself—even out loud—why you're feeling down or negative at a particular moment, then take full responsibility for addressing the issue(s) at hand. Stop when you feel like you're spinning out of control and ask yourself the following questions that will help you get inside your mind:

- What am I aware of?
- What am I feeling?
- What am I thinking about?
- What do I want?

Interconnectedness. Think about how you move in this world, and how your energy affects others. Identify with people and things!

Innovation. Be creative. Keep a journal or take a class. Make it a point to do things in a better or more efficient way. Question established information and challenge conventional wisdom. More importantly, move away from stasis, towards growth. HBV can't stand that.

IN A SENTENCE:

> *HBV is both a challenge and a gift, and we can feel proud about how much we've learned and grown this year.*

Resources

Hepatitis B Antigens/Antibody Cheat Sheet

NAME	DEFINITION	ALSO KNOWN AS
HBeAg	Hepatitis B e antigen	Envelope antigen
HBsAg	Hepatitis B surface antigen	Surface antigen, Australian antigen
HBcAg	Hepatitis B core antigen	Core antigen
HBeAb	Hepatitis B e antibody	Anti-HBe
HBsAb	Hepatitis B surface antibody	Anti-HBs
HBcAb	Hepatitis B core antibody	Anti-HBc
Anti-HBcIgM	M class immunoglobulin antibody to hepatitis B core antigen (shows recent infection)	IgM Anti-HBc, IgM antibody to HBcAg
Anti-HBcIgG	G class immunoglobulin antibody to hepatitis B core antigen (shows past infection)	IgG Anti Hbc
HBV DNA	Viral load	Hep B Virus, HBV
HBiG	Hepatitis B immunoglobulin	

My Lab Results

DATE	MM/YY	MM/YY	MM/YY	MM/YY	MM/YY	MM/YY
ALT–Alanine transaminase (SGPT)						
AST–Aspartate aminotransferase (SGOT)						
HBV DNA–Viral Load						
LDH–Lactate dehydrogenase						
ALP–Alkaline phosphatase						
GGT–Gamma-glutamyl transpeptidase						
Total Bilirubin–Direct and Indirect						
Bilirubin–urine–Direct bilirubin-urine						
Albumin						
TP–Total Protein						
PT/INR						
PTT–Partial thromboplastin time						
WBC white blood cells						
Platelets–Platelet/thrombocyte count						
AFP–Alpha FetoProtein						
TIBC–Total iron binding capacity						
Ferritin						
Cholesterol						
Uric Acid						

My Lab Results (continued)

DATE	MM/YY	MM/YY	MM/YY	MM/YY	MM/YY	MM/YY
Sodium						
Potassium						
Chloride						
CO$_2$–Carbon dioxide						
BUN–Blood urea nitrogen						
Creatine						
Hemoglobin						
HGB–Hgb electrophoresis						
TSH–Thyroid stimulating hormone						
HBsAg						
HBsAb						
HBeAg						
HBeAb						
Anti-HCV Ab						
Anti-Delta Ab						
HIV						
Testosterone						
Endoscopy/Grade of varices						
Ultrasound						

Biopsy Grading and Staging

The following are abridged versions of the various grading scales currently in use for liver biopsies. Your biopsy report will use one or more of the following:

HAI

Knodell (1981)
    I.   Periportal +/-bridging necrosis (Score 0–6)
    II.   Intralobular degeneration and focal necrosis (Score 0–4)
    III. Portal inflammation (Score 0–4)
    IV. Fibrosis (Score 0–4)

Ludwig (1993)
    I—Portal and Lobular Inflammatory Activity Grade 0–4
    II—Fibrosis
    Stage 1-3
    Stage 4 Probable or definite cirrhosis

Ishak (1995)
Necroinflammatory Scores
A. *Periportal (piecemeal necrosis)*
    0 = Absent
    1 = Mild (focal, few portal areas)
    2 = Mild/moderate (focal, most portal areas)
    3 = Moderate around <50% of tracts or septa)
    4 = Severe (continuous around >50% of tracts or septa)

B. *Confluent necrosis*
    0 = Absent
    1 = Focal confluent necrosis
    2 Zone 3 necrosis in some areas
    3 Zone 3 necrosis in most areas
    4 Zone 3 necrosis, plus occasional portal-central (P-C) bridging
    5 Zone 3 necrosis, plus multiple P-C bridging Panacinar or multiacinar necrosis

C. *Focal (spotty) necrosis and focal inflammation*
    0—Absent
    1—One focus or less per high power field (HPF)
    2—Two to four foci per HPF

3—Five to ten foci per HPF
4—More than ten foci HPF

D. Portal inflammation

0—None
1—Mild, some or all portal areas
2—Moderate, some or all portal areas
3—Moderate/marked, all portal areas
4—Marked, all portal areas

E. Architectural Changes: Fibrosis/Cirrhosis

0 = No fibrosis
1 = Fibrous expansion of some portal areas
2 = Fibrous expansion of most portal areas
3 = Fibrous expansion of most portal areas with occasional portal to portal bridging
4 = Fibrous expansion of portal areas with marked bridging
5 = Marked bridging with occasional nodules (incomplete cirrhosis)
6 = Cirrhosis, probable or definite

For Further Information

THE FOLLOWING resources and recommended publications were very helpful in writing this book. For more in-depth information, please consult the following sources:

National and International Organizations

Hepatitis B Foundation
700 East Butler Avenue
Doylestown, PA 18901-2697
(215) 489-4900
www.hepb.org/

American Liver Foundation
1425 Pompton Avenue
Cedar Grove, NJ 07009-1000
(201) 256-2550 (800-GO-LIVER)
www.liverfoundation.org/

Hepatitis Foundation International
30 Sunrise Terrace
Cedar Grove, NJ 07009-1423
(800) 324-7305
www.hepfi.org/

**Bill and Melinda Gates Children's
  Vaccine Program**
4 Nickerson Street
Seattle, WA 98109-1699
(206) 285-3500
info@childrensvaccine.org
www.childrensvaccine.org

Immunization Action Coalition
1573 Selby Avenue, Suite 234
St. Paul, MN 55104
(651) 647-9009
admin@immunize.org
http://www.immunize.org/

World Health Organization
Avenue Appia 20
1211 Geneva 27
Switzerland
+00 41 22 791 21 11
info@who.int
www.who.int/home-page/

**Centers for Disease Control,
  Hepatitis Branch**
Mailstop A33
National Center for Infectious Diseases (NCID)
1600 Clifton Road N.E.
Atlanta, GA 30333
(888) 443-7232
www.cdc.gov/ncidod/diseases/hepatitis

Gay and Lesbian Medical Association (GLMA)
459 Fulton Street, Suite 107
San Francisco, CA 94102
(415) 255-4547
info@glma.org
www.glma.org/home.html

National Kidney Foundation
30 East 33rd Street
New York, NY 10016
(800) 622-9010
Provides information for people with hepatitis C and/or hepatitis B who are on renal dialysis.

American College of Gastroenterology
4900 B South 31st Street
Arlington, VA 22206
(800) 978-7666 Hotline
www.acg.gi.org

National Women's Health Network
514 10th Street NW, Suite 400
Washington, DC 20004
(202) 347-1140
For health information:
(202) 628-7814
www.womenshealthnetwork.org/

Latino Organization for Liver Awareness (LOLA)
Debbie Delgado-Vega, Founder and CEO
P.O. Box 842
Throggs Neck Station,
Bronx, NY 10465
(718) 892-8697
(888) 367-LOLA
www.lola-national.org/

National Coalition of Hispanic Health and Human Services Organizations
1501 16th Street, NW
Washington, DC 20036
(202) 797-4353
www.hispanichealth.org/

Office of Minority Health Resource Center
PO Box 37337
Washington, DC 20013-7337
(800) 444-6472

Government Resources

Center for Disease Control (CDC)
1600 Clifton Road, NE
Atlanta, GA 30333
(404) 332-4555
www.cdc.gov/

Disability Rights Section, Civil Rights Division
United States Department of Justice
PO Box 66738
Washington, DC 20035-6738
(800) 514-0301

Equal Employment Opportunity Commission (EEOC)
JFK Federal Building Government Center
4th Floor, Room 475
Boston, MA 02203
(617) 565-3190

Medicare
(800) 633-4227
www.medicare.gov

National Center for Complementary and Alternative Medicine Clearinghouse
PO Box 8218
Silver Spring, MD 2907-8218
(888) 644-6226
(800) 325-0778 (TTY)
www.nccam.nih.gov/

Social Security Administration
Office of Public Inquiries
6401 Security Boulevard
Room 4-C-5 Annex
Baltimore, MD 21235-6401
(800) 772-1213
www.ssa.gov/

USDA Food and Nutrition Information Center
Agricultural Research Service, USDA
National Agricultural Library, Room 105
10301 Baltimore Avenue
Beltsville, MD 20705-2351
(301) 504-5719
(301) 504-6856 (TTY)
fnic@nal.usda.gov
www.nal.usda.gov/fnic

U.S. Department of Labor
Family Medical Leave Act
www.dol.gov/dol/esa/fmla.htm

Drug and Alcohol Resources

Alcoholics Anonymous World Services (AA)
475 Riverside Drive
New York, NY 10163
(212) 870-3400

Drug Abuse Information and Treatment Referral Line
National Institute on Drug Abuse
11426 Rockville Pike, Suite 410
Rockville, MD 20852
(800) 662-4357
(800) 662-9832 (Spanish)
(800) 228-0427 (hearing impaired)

Narcotics Anonymous
(818) 773-9999
www.na.org

National Clearinghouse for Alcohol and Drug Information
PO Box 100
Summit, NJ 07901-0100
(800) 262-2463

Exercise

American Council on Exercise (ACE)
4851 Paramount Drive
San Diego, California 92123
(800) 825-3636
www.acefitness.org/

American Yoga Association
PO Box 19986
Sarasota, FL 34276
(941) 927-4977
www.americanyogaassociation.org

Hot Lines

GENERAL
Hepatitis Help Line:
(800) 390-1202

STD (Sexually Transmitted Diseases) National Hot Line:
(800) 227-8922

MINORITY ISSUES
Association of Asian-Pacific Community Health Organizations:
(510) 272-9536

National Coalition of Hispanic Health and Human Services Organization:
(202) 387-5000

The Office of Minority Health Resource Center:
(800) 444-6472

WOMEN'S ISSUES
National Women's Health Resource Center:
(202) 537-4015

Publications

B-Informed
Free newsletter of the Hepatitis B Foundation
(215) 489-4900
www.hepb.org

Hepatitis Magazine
523 N. Sam Houston Parkway East
Suite 300
Houston, TX 77060
(281) 272-2744
www.hepatitismag.com

Hepatology
Journal of the American Association for the Study of Liver Disease
W.B. Saunders Company
PO Box 628239
Orlando, FL 32862-8239
(800) 654-2452
http://customerservice.wbsaunders.com (for subscription information)
http://hepatology.aasldjournals.org

Progress
Newsletter of the American Liver Foundation
(800) GO-LIVER
www.liverfoundation.org

Websites

PHARMACEUTICAL COMPANIES:
Bristol-Myers Squibb
www.bms.com

Gilead Sciences
www.gilead.com

GlaxoSmithKline
www.gsk.com
www.worldwidevaccines.com/public/
diseas/hepb3.asp

Sciclone Pharmaceuticals
www.sciclone.com

Schering Plough
www.schering.com

Hepatitis-specific sites

HBV Adoption Support Group
http://groups.yahoo.com/group/hbv-adoption

Health Central
www.healthcentral.com

Hepatitis Central
www.hepatitis-central.com

Hepatitis Neighborhood
www.hepatitisneighborhood.com/

HepNet, the Hepatitis Information Network
www.hepnet.com

Hepatitis Magazine
(800) 310-7047
www.hepatitismag.com

HIV and Hepatitis Treatment Advocates
www.hivandhepatitis.com/

Medline
www.nlm.nih.org

Medscape
www.medscape.com

WebMD
http://my.webmd.com/

National Library of Medicine
www.nlm.nih.gov
(888) FIND-NLM

Organ donation

United Network for Organ Sharing (UNOS)
National Transplantation Resource Center
1100 Boulders Parkway, Suite 500

PO Box 13770
Richmond, VA 23225-8770
www.unos.org
librarian@unos.org
(804) 330-8546

Related diseases

AFSA, Inc.
The American Fibromyalgia Syndrome Association, Inc.
6380 E. Tanque Verde, Suite D
Tucson, AZ 85715
(520) 733-1570
www.afsafund.org/

Alternative Medicine

National Center for Homeopathy
801 North Fairfax Street, Suite 306
Alexandria, VA 22314
(703) 548-7790
www.homeopathic.org

American Foundation of Traditional Chinese Medicine
505 Beach Street
San Francisco, CA 94133
(415) 776-0502

Institute for Traditional Medicine
2017 SE Hawthorne
Portland, OR 97214
www.itmonline.org/

American Association of Oriental Medicine (AAOM)
433 Front Street
Catasauqua, PA 18032
(610) 266-1433
www.aaom.org

American Holistic Health Association (AHHA)
Department R
PO Box 17400
Anaheim, CA 92817-7400
(714) 779-6152
http://ahha.org

Ayurvedic Institute
11311 Menaul NE
Albuquerque, New Mexico 78112
(505) 291-9698
www.ayurveda.com

Glossary

ACUTE: A descriptor that denotes the abrupt onset of a disease or an abnormal condition lasting a short amount of time; a disease is termed "acute" in comparison to a "chronic disease," which may persist indefinitely or without change. Acute viral hepatitis is a sudden and short-term inflammation of the liver—i.e., acute HBV appears between 4 to 32 weeks after exposure, though, 90–95 percent of individuals infected will recover completely.

ACUPUNCTURE: The treatment of pain or disease by inserting the tips of needles at specific points on the skin.

ACUTE VIRAL HEPATITIS: See acute.

ADEFOVIR: See nucleoside analogues.

AFLATOXINS: A toxin produced by the fungus Aspergillus flavus, which is often found in improperly stored grains and peanuts. Aflatoxins can cause hepatocellular carcinoma.

ALBUMIN: A protein that is formed in the liver and excreted by the kidneys. Liver disease causes a decrease in albumin, which can lead to ascites or edema.

ALKALINE PHOSPHATASE (ALP): An enzyme that is found in bacteria, fungi, and animals but not in higher plants. In humans, ALP is found in the liver, biliary tract, bones, and the placenta. High levels of ALP indicate bone growth, bile obstruction, or liver disease. High levels of ALP are a warning sign of cirrhosis.

ALPHA INTERFERON: See Interferon.

AMERICANS WITH DISABILITIES ACT (ADA): The U.S. law, enacted 1990, which protects the civil rights of individuals with disabilities in the same way that individuals' civil rights are protected on the basis of race, color, sex, national origin, age, and religion. This act guarantees equal opportunity for individuals with disabilities in public accommodations, employment, transportation, state and local government services, and telecommunications. It is important for an individual with HBV to be aware of her/his civil rights in the workplace—employment based on one's HBV condition can be legally protected. See the Americans with Disabilities Act website for further explanation: www.usdoj.gov/crt/ada/adahom1.htm.

AMINO ACID: Any one of a class of simple organic compounds containing carbon, hydrogen, oxygen, nitrogen, and, in certain cases, sulfur. These compounds are the building blocks of proteins. Following the digestion of food proteins, amino acids are released into the intestinal tract and carried in the bloodstream to the body cells, where they are used for growth, maintenance, and repair.

AMINOTRANSFERASE: An enzyme that modifies proteins. The two aminotransferases important in hepatology are aspartate aminotransferase (AST) and alanine aminotransferase (ALT). As a general practice, doctors run blood tests that track their patient's ALT and AST counts as a way to gauge the inflammation of her/his liver.

ANAMNESTIC RESPONSE: From the Greek "to recall." A response in which the immune system remembers an antigen and subsequently creates antibodies to fight it, even if many years since vaccination or previous infection.

ANTIBODY: A three-lobed globulin that contains two short and two long chains of protein found in the blood or other bodily fluids. Antibodies are stimulated by the presence of antigens, over which it has a destructive influence.

ANTICOAGULANT: Any substance that prevents the coagulation of blood.

ANTIGEN: Any material (proteins, toxins, microorganisms, or tissue cells) capable of triggering in a person the production of specific antibodies or the formation of lymphocytes, which react with the particular material. A material is an antigen in an individual depending on the dose of the material or whether it's foreign to her/his genetic makeup.

ANTIOXIDANTS: Enzymes or other organic substances, such as vitamins C, E, and beta-carotene that are capable of counteracting the damaging effects of oxidation in healthy cells and tissue. Antioxidants rid the body of harmful atoms called free radicals that circulate an individual's system and damage molecules. Since HBV causes one to have more free radicals, antioxidants, such as lipoic acid, glutathione and limonene, are a recommended dietary supplement for detoxifying the liver.

ARTHRALGIA: Neuralgic pain in a joint or joints.

ASCITES: (pronounced as-SY-tees) The accumulation of free serous (watery) fluid in the abdominal cavity in clinically detectable amounts, which occur as a result of cirrhosis, kidney failure, and congestive heart failure.

ASPARTATE TRANSAMINASE (AST): An enzyme that is released into blood circulation after the injury or death of cells. The amount of AST in the blood directly corresponds to the number of damaged cells. Accordingly, doctors examine their patients' AST levels as a way to detect a variety of diseases, among them cirrhosis and alcoholic hepatitis.

ASSAY: A qualitative or quantitative analysis of a substance, i.e., the amount of HBV in blood.

ASYMPTOMATIC: A person who does not show symptoms. Chronic HBV is almost entirely asymptomatic, which is the reason why the condition often goes undetected in individual carriers.

AUTOIMMUNE HEPATITIS: A type of hepatitis characterized by tissue injury that results from a person's immunologic reaction with her/his own tissues.

AYURVEDA: The ancient Hindu science of health and medicine.

BASELINE: The basis for subsequent measurement. In HBV, baseline is determined by the first tests you do after initial diagnosis.

BILE: A bitter yellowish-brown or brownish-green liquid secreted by the liver and stored in the gallbladder. Bile aids digestion by emulsifying fats.

BILIRUBIN: An orange-red pigment created from hemoglobin during the destruction of erythrocytes (a type of red blood cell) in the presence of liver disease. Accumulation of bilirubin causes jaundice.

BILIARY TRACT: The ducts that drain bile from the liver to the intestine.

BIOPSY (LIVER): The removal and examination of liver tissue from the living body for the purpose of diagnosis. An HBV patient may be asked to undergo a liver biopsy as a way to gauge the severity and extent of scarring that occurs due to her/his infection.

BLOOD UREA NITROGEN (BUN): A term primarily used in reference to the medical test that evaluates renal (kidney) function. BUN, however, may also indicate liver disease or dehydration.

CARBOHYDRATES: Any of the group of organic compounds composed of carbon, hydrogen, and oxygen, such as sugars, starches, and cellulose. Carbohydrates are essential fuel for individuals' energy, comprising more than half of the calories needed in a balanced diet.

CATECHIN: A bioflavonoid (a vitamin) found in green tea that has both antiviral and antioxidant qualities. Catechin is a demonstrated treatment of viral hepatitis as well as a preventative treatment of oxidative damage to the heart, kidney, lungs, and spleen.

cccDNA (COVALENTLY CLOSED CIRCULAR DNA): HBV forms a tight "supercoil" of closed circular DNA in order to be transported into the nucleus of the liver cell.

CHOLESTATIC LIVER DISEASE: Cholestatic liver diseases such as primary biliary cirrhosis (PBC) and primary sclerosing cholangitis (PSC) are characterized by destruction of bile ducts leading to cholestasis, inflammation, fibrosis, and eventually cirrhosis.

CHOLESTEROL: A white, waxy crystalline organic alcohol present in animal fats, oils, bile, brain tissue, blood, and egg yolk. In humans, the liver manufactures cholesterol and simultaneously removes it via tiny receptors in liver cells. High levels of cholesterol in blood (from high-fat food intake) can clog the receptors, causing cholesterol levels to rise and, thus, make individuals (particularly those with HBV) more susceptible to other health complications.(e.g., eye, kidney, and nerve disease).

CHRONIC: A descriptor denoting a slow-progressing disease that persists over a long period. A disease is termed "chronic" in comparison to an "acute disease," which may have a rapid onset and short duration.

CIRRHOSIS: A chronic disease of the liver marked by diffuse, irreversible fibrosis, which interferes with liver functioning and circulation.

COAGULOPATHY: A disease that affects the blood-clotting process.

CO-INFECTED: A term that indicates the invasion in a person's body of more than one virus. It is not uncommon, particularly in developing countries, for individuals to be co-infected by HIV and HBV.

COLLAGEN: The supportive protein component of connective tissue, bone, cartilage, and skin. Damage to hepatocytes as a result of HBV destroys the collagen that circulates around and between liver cells, thus, eventuating in fibrosis.

COMPUTERIZED TOMOGRAPHY (CT): See tomography.

CREATININE: A protein that is produced by creatinine metabolism. Creatinine is normally released into the blood at a constant rate. The clearance rate of creatinine is indicative of the regular functioning of one's kidneys. Thus, creatinine also refers to a blood test that is conducted (usually before a biopsy) to gauge the severity of HBV infection.

CYANOSIS: Blue discoloration of the lips due to severe cirrhosis.

DANDELION: A perennial herb of the genus Taraxacum of the family Asteraceae. Historically, dandelions have been cultivated both as medicine and food by traditional Chinese, Ayurvedic, and Western practices. Dandelions have anti-inflammatory and hepatotonic effects.

DECOMPENSATION: The failure of one's liver to compensate for damage or injury, resulting in a decrease of liver functions.

DNA (DEOXYRIBONUCLEIC ACID): The molecular base of heredity that is present in chromosomes. DNA is responsible for the replication of the key substances of life: proteins and nucleic acid.

E ANTIGEN: See antigen.

EDEMA: Swelling of the legs. Edema is one possible symptom of severe liver disease.

ENCEPHALOPATHY: Any disease of the brain, also known as cerebopathy. Encephalopathy is an urgent marker of fulminant hepatitis.

ENDOSCOPY: The inspection of an internal cavity or air and food passage by using an endoscope (medical instrument for conducting this procedure). HBV patients often undergo gastrointestinal endoscopy procedures as a way to detect varices.

ENGERIX-B : See vaccine.

ENTECAVIR: See nucleoside analogues.

ENZYME: A protein secreted by the body, which initiates or accelerates a chemical change in another substance while remaining unchanged in the process. Liver enzymes, in particular, are produced by the liver. In HBV patients, an elevated liver enzyme count often indicates hepatocytic necrosis, a condition caused by chronic hepatitis.

EPITOPES: The site on the surface of an antigen molecule to which a particular antibody (produced by the immune system) attaches itself.

EPIDEMIOLOGY: The factors that control the presence or absence of a disease or pathogen.

FIBROSIS: The formation of fibrous tissue. Fibrosis is a distinct indication of an abnormal degenerative process (i.e., HBV). Severe fibrosis or cirrhosis can cause varicose (dilated) veins.

FOOD AND DRUG ADMINISTRATION (FDA): An agency of the Public Health Service division of the U.S. Department of Health and Human Services. The FDA was created to protect public health by ensuring that foods are safe and pure, cosmetics and other chemical substances are harmless, and products are safe, effective, and honestly labeled. The FDA also ensures prior-evidence-of-safety tests and procedures for new drugs, pesticides as well as additives and colorings in foods and cosmetics.

FTC (COVARICIL): See nucleoside analogues.

FULMINANT HEPATITIS B: A rapidly progressive form of hepatitis with necrosis of large areas of the liver.

GAMMA GLUTAMYLTANSERASE (GGT): An enzyme present in the kidney, liver, and pancreas. The consumption of alcoholic beverages elevates an individual's GGT levels; thus, GGT is a useful marker of alcohol intake and alcohol-induced liver disease.

GASTROINTESTINAL: A term that denotes relation to the stomach and the intestines.

GASTROINTESTINAL ENDOSCOPY: See endoscopy.

GENE THERAPY: The introduction of a functional gene into an organism as a way to replace or supplement the activity of a defective one.

GENOTYPE: The genetic variation of an HBV virus.

GIANOTTI-CROSTI SYNDROME: Cutaneous (pertaining to the skin) manifestation of HBV infection that results from an eruption of papules (solid elevation of the skin) on one's arms and face. This skin condition will typically disappear within thirty to sixty days.

GINGER: A member of the *Zingiberaceae* family of tropical and subtropical perennial herbs. Adopting the thousand-year Chinese tradition of using the herb as a natural treatment for nausea, HBV patients have found that taking ginger (usually in the form of tea) relieves nausea induced by chemotherapy treatments.

GINSENG: A member of the *Araliaceae* family of tropical herbs, shrubs, and trees, which are valuable for their medicinal qualities, in particular, for regulating blood and sugar levels and stimulating sexual desire. HBV patients find that ginseng effectively relieves mental fatigue (i.e., brain fog) and functions as an immunomodulator (a treatment that strengthens the immune system).

GLOSSITIS: Inflammation of the tongue.

GLUTATHIONE: See antioxidants.

GYNECOMASTIA: Development of breasts in men due to cirrhosis-related hormonal imbalance.

HBV MARKERS: See marker.

HEMODIALYSIS: The removal of waste materials or poisons from blood by means of a hemodialyzer (artificial kidney apparatus). Historically, hemodialysis has been a significant route of transmission for HBV.

HEMOGLOBIN: A respiratory protein found in the erythrocytes (red blood cells) of all vertebrates (any animal with a backbone or spinal column) and some invertebrates. Hemoglobin also refers to a blood test (usually given before a biopsy) to gauge the severity of HBV infection.

HEMOLYSIS: A breakdown of red blood cells.

HEPATITIS: Inflammation of and damage to the liver.

HEPATOCELLULAR CARCINOMA (HCC): A malignant hepatocellular tumor that first invades the tissue of the liver, eventually spreads to other parts of the body and, ultimately, leads to death. Chronic active HBV eventuates in HCC.

HEPATOCYTE: A liver cell.

HEPATOCYTE NECROSIS: See **necrosis**.

HEPATOLOGIST: A doctor who specializes in diseases of the liver (e.g., hepatitis).

HEPATOLOGY: The study of the liver and its diseases (e.g., hepatitis).

HISTOLOGICAL ACTIVITY INDEX (HAI): A formulaic indicator of hepatocellular necrosis, fibrosis, and cirrhosis. Doctors use HAI (also known as Knodell's Index) as a way to determine, or judge the effectiveness of, an HBV treatment.

HOLISTIC HEALTH: An expanded definition of healing that puts emphasis on the whole person (body, mind, and spirit).

HOMEOPATHY: A treatment strategy developed in the 1800s with the simple idea that "like cures like." Highly diluted quantities of substances—herbs, chemicals, minerals, and animal products—are thought to reverse the symptoms of disease that they, in turn, induce.

HUMAN IMMUNODEFICIENCY VIRUS (HIV): A virus that is characterized by active virus replication and progressive immunologic impairment and, ultimately, causes AIDS (Acquired Immune Deficiency Syndrome). HIV also indicates that a person is infected by a strain of the Human Immunodeficiency Virus.

HYDROGENATION: A process that changes liquid oil, naturally high in unsaturated fat, to a more solid and saturated form. As a general rule, the greater the degree of hydrogenation, the more saturated the fat becomes. There is great misunderstanding and debate about the effect of hydrogenation upon the composition and nutritional properties of edible fats and oils. Recent studies, though, suggest that fats that have undergone the hydrogenation process may raise blood cholesterol.

HYPERTENSION/PORTAL HYPERTENSION: The existence of high arterial blood pressure in adults usually defined as pressures exceeding 140/90 mmHg. Many HBV patients suffer from hypertension, which results from fibrosis in the blood channels of the liver.

IMMUNIZATION: The act or process by which a person becomes resistant or immune to a harmful agent (e.g., a virus). An individual can be immunized against the hepatitis virus by receiving the hepatitis vaccine treatment.

IMMUNOGLOBULIN: A protein molecule functioning as a specific antibody, which has two main functions: to bind to an antigen or to mediate the binding of molecules to host tissues.

IMMUNOMODULATARY: Describing any of various methods of therapeutic manipulation of the body's immune response to an antigen.

INCUBATION PERIOD: The period between initial contact with the virus and the first appearance of HBV markers

INTERFERON: A protein substance produced by body cells in response to invasion by viruses which literally interferes with the synthesis of new viruses. Alpha Interferon, marketed by the pharmaceutical corporation Schering-Plough as a treatment for HBV, is a synthetic version of the naturally produced Interferon in a person's body. A few Interferon drugs currently on the market are Intron A, Roferon, and Inergen.

INTERNATIONAL UNITS PER LITER (IU/L): A metric system that measures volume. Blood tests are often expressed in IU/L's.

JAUNDICE: The yellow pigmentation of skin and/or sclera (the white membraneous part of an eye) caused by high levels of bilirubin in the blood.

KNODELL'S INDEX: See **Histological Activity Index**.

LAMIVUDINE: A nucleoside analogue treatment that was originally manufactured by the pharmaceutical corporation GlaxoSmithKline. The drug is also known as Epivir, 3TC, or Zeffix.

LAPAROSCOPY: A procedure that allows visualization of the contents of the abdominal cavity by means of an endoscope. This technique is used for conducting a biopsy, in particular, on patients with advanced liver disease or complications with bleeding.

LICHEN PLANUS: An eruption of flat papules (solid elevations) with depressed purplish centers on the skin.

LICORICE ROOT: A European plant, *Glycyrrhiza glabra,* of the *Leguminosae* family that is cultivated for its medicinal properties, typically, for coughs and constipation. However, licorice root also has antiviral and anti-inflammatory properties in addition to its function as an immunomodulator (a treatment that strengthens the immune system).

LIMONINE: See **antioxidants**.

LIPOIC ACID: See **antioxidants**.

LIPOPROTEINS: A conjugated protein containing fat as the non-protein substance. Low-density lipoproteins are responsible for most of the cholesterol deposits in arteries.

LIVER: A large dark red gland that produces and secretes bile and plays an important role in the metabolism of carbohydrates, fats, protein, minerals, and vitamins. The liver is the largest glandular organ (a secreting organ) in the body. The hepatitis virus causes inflammation of the liver.

LIVER FUNCTION TESTS (LFTs): Medical tests that measure the antigens and antibodies in a person's blood.

LIVER TRANSPLANT: The transplantation of a liver in cases of irreversible, progressive liver disease.

LOW-DENSITY LIPOPROTEIN (LDL): See **lipoprotein**.

LYMPHOCYTE: A white blood cell formed in the lymnoid tissue; a.k.a., a lymph cell.

MARKER: A term referring to the positive and negative symbols appearing on a person's blood test results, which indicate the presence of antigens or antibodies in her/his blood. A marker is also a term used by doctors to help explain or gauge a disorder.

MASTITIS: Inflammation of the breast.

MEDEVA: See **vaccine**.

MEDIUM CHAIN TRIGLYCERIDE (MCT): A class of fatty acids found in coconut oil and butter. MCTs are differentiated from other fats because they have a slightly lower calorie content and are absorbed and burned rapidly as energy—a quality that resembles carbohydrates rather than fats.

MILK THISTLE: A member of the *Compositae* family of annual or biennial herbs, *Silybum marianum,* which grow up to 6 feet tall bearing prickly edged leaves streaked with conspicuous white veins and crimson flowers. The seeds, fruit, and leaves of milk thistle have been used since the Roman era as a liver tonic. Numerous clinical studies prove the therapeutic effects of the plant for treating several types of liver ailments such as cirrhosis, chronic hepatitis, and fatty infiltration of the liver.

NECROSIS: The death of bodily tissue in a circumscribed area. Hepatocellular necrosis, in particular, is the localized tissue death of hepatic (liver) cells.

NUCLEOSIDE ANALOGUES: A class of drugs that interferes with HBV replication.

PCR (POLYMERASE CHAIN REACTION): A highly sophisticated blood test that measures the amount of HBV DNA in your blood.

PEGYLATED INTERFERON: A newer kind of interferon that is time-released thanks to a gellike substance called polyethylene glycol. Pegylated Interferon allows patients to limit the number of weekly injections to just one, and may help mitigate more severe side effects.

PERCUTANEOUS BIOPSY: See **biopsy.**

PERINATAL TRANSMISSION: Transmission of a disease from mother to child.

PERITONITIS: Inflammation of the peritoneum (the serous membrane lining the wall of the abdominal and pelvic cavities) that is marked by pain, fever, and constipation, and caused by bacterial infection, e.g., escaped bile. Peritonitis is a common medical consequence of a complicated liver biopsy, which often results from (about 1 percent of the time) a punctured gallbladder.

PHYLLANTHUS AMARUS: A flowering perennial herb, *Phyllantus amanes,* that has been used in traditional Asian medical practices as a diuretic and antiseptic, as well as for relieving diarrhea and general stomach pains. Scientists have found antihepatitis B surface antigen activity in the herb in controlled studies.

PLATELET: A disk-shaped, colorless proto-plasmic structure that is present in the blood of mammals. Platelets play an important role in blood coagulation. Normal levels for humans range between 150,000 to 300,000 platelets per mm^3. For individuals with HBV, the presence of platelets markedly decreases after the progression of cirrhosis. Thus, platelet count often refers to a blood test (usually given before a biopsy) to gauge the severity of HBV infection.

PLATELET COUNT: See **platelet**.

POLYMERASE CHAIN REACTION: A laboratory process in which a particular DNA segment from a mixture of DNA chains is rapidly replicated, thus, producing a large, readily analyzed sample piece of DNA.

POLYPEPTIDE: A peptide (compound which contains two or more amino acids linked by the carboxyl group of one amino acid to the amino group of another) containing many molecules of amino acids.

PORTAL HYPERTENSION: See **hypertension**.

PRECORE MUTANT HBV: A strain of HBV that evolves without the assistance of HBeAg.

PROTEINS: Any of a group of nitrogeneous substances of high molecular weight that contain amino acids as their fundamental structural unit, are present in cells of all animals and plants, and function in all phases of the chemical and physical activity of cells.

PROTHROMBIN TIME INTERNATIONAL NORMALIZED RATIO (PTT) OR PARTIAL THROMBOPLASTIN TIME (PT): A blood test (usually given before a biopsy) that measures the time it takes for blood to clot. This is important for HBV patients because liver cell damage and bile flow obstruction (two consequences of HBV) interfere with the blood clotting process.

PRURITIS: Persistent and severe itching of clinically normal skin that results from systemic disease. Pruritis is a common symptom of HBV.

RNA (RIBONUCLEIC ACID): Any of a family of polymacleotides (a component of all living cells).

SCHIZANDRA: A flowering vine, Schizandrae chinensis produces white flowers and bunches of small red berries. In traditional Asian medical practices (specifically in China and Russia), schizandra is used as a treatment for asthma, coughing and other respiratory problems, diarrhea, insomnia, impotence, and complications of the liver. In clinical trials, schizandra has lowered ALT levels in an average of 90 percent of research participants.

SEROCONVERSION: A change in immunologic reactivity of the serum (watery fluid) from negative to positive for a particular antibody.

SERUM GLUTANIC-OXALOACETIC: See aminotransferase.

SERUM GLUTANIC-PYRUVIC TRANSAMINASE: See aminotransferase.

SPIDER NEVI: Spidery red veins that appear on the upper body, arms, and face as a result of portal hypertension and cirrhosis.

SUPERINFECTION: A condition in which one viral infection is superimposed on another preexisting viral infection.

TITRES: The highest dilution of a material (in particular, serum) that produces a reaction in the immunologic test system.

TOMOGRAPHY: The radiography of a selected level of the body. Doctors use computerized tomography (tomography using a computer-assisted tomograph) to help determine the best point of entry for the biopsy needle.

ULTRASOUND: A medical technique that uses sound waves to study and treat hard-to-reach areas of the body. Ultrasound is noninvasive, involves no radiation, and avoids the possible hazards such as bleeding, infection, or reactions to chemicals typical of other diagnostic methods.

UREA: The principal product of protein metabolism. The liver produces nontoxic urea by converting amino acids and compounds of ammonia so that these compounds can pass through the bodily system.

VACCINE: A preparation of dead or live attenuated viruses or bacteria, which induces in a person active immunity to infectious disease. The HBV vaccine, available since 1981, is used to prevent contraction of, and, ultimately, to eradicate, the hepatitis B virus.

VARICES: Dilated veins. Varices develop in the esophagus and stomach as a result of cirrhosis (a consequence of long-term HBV infection).

VARICOSE VEINS: Abnormally dilated and tortuous veins that develop as a result of liver scarring.

VIRAL LOAD: The amount of virus in your blood. This quantity is expressed in copies per milliliter of blood.

VIRUS: An intracellular, infectious parasite that can only survive and reproduce in living cells. Each virus particle is composed of a protein shell that encloses a single nucleic acid, either RNA or DNA. The Hepatitis B virus is a DNA virus from the *Hepadnoviridae* family.

YMDD: A region on the viral polymerase of HBV where Lamivudine has its action and where resistance develops. The incidence of YMDD Lamivudine resistance increases with duration of therapy.

For Further Reading

General Guides on Liver Disorders

Chopra, Sanjiv, M.D. *Dr. Sanjiv Chopra's Liver Book: A Comprehensive Guide to Diagnosis, Treatment and Recovery*. New York: Pocket Books, 2001.

Palmer, Melissa, M.D. *Guide to Hepatitis and Liver Disease: What You Need to Know*. Garden City Park, NJ: Avery Publishing Group, 1999.

Schiff, Eugene R., Michael F. Sorrell, and Willis C. Maddrey, eds. *Schiff's Diseases of the Liver on CD-ROM*. Philadelphia: Lippincott Williams & Wilkins Publishers, 1998.

Clinical Focus

Blumberg, Baruch. *Hepatitis B and the Prevention of Cancer of the Liver: Selected Publications of Baruch S. Blumberg*. River Edge, NJ: World Scientific, 2000.

Blumberg, Baruch. *Hepatitis B: The Hunt for a Killer Virus*. Princeton, NJ: Princeton University Press, 2002.

Ellis, Richard W. *Hepatitis B Vaccines in Clinical Practice*. New York: Marcel Dekker, 1992.

Muraskin, William. *The War Against Hepatitis B: A History of the International Task Force on Hepatitis B Immunization*. Philadelphia: University of Pennsylvania Press, 1995.

Schiff, Eugene R., Willis C. Maddrey, and Michael F. Sorrell, eds. *Transplantation of the Liver*. Philadelphia: Lippincott Williams & Wilkins Publishers, 2000

Hepatology Textbooks and Journals

Bircher, J., ed. *Oxford Textbook of Clinical Hepatology*, 2nd edition. Oxford, England: Oxford University Press, 1999.

Rodés, J., ed. *Journal of Hepatology*. Oxford, England: Elsevier Science 2001.

Zakim, David and Thomas Boyer, eds. *Hepatology: A Textbook of Liver Disease*, 3rd edition. St. Louis, MO: W.B. Saunders Co., 1996.

Guides and Texts on Hepatitis B

Blumberg, Baruch. *Hepatitis B and the Prevention of Cancer of the Liver: Selected Publications of Baruch S. Blumberg*. Princeton, NJ: World Scientific Publishing Company, Incorporated, 1997.

Everson, Gregory T. and Hedy Weinberg. *Living with Hepatitis B*. New York: The Hatherleigh Company, Limited, 2002.

Maddrey, Willis C., M.D. and Eugene R. Schiff, M.D. *Be in Charge, A Guide to Living with Chronic Hepatitis B and C*. Kenilworth, NJ: Schering Corporation, 1998. (booklet)

Millman, Irving. *Hepatitis B: The Virus, the Disease and the Vaccine*. Reading, MA: Perseus, 1984.

Herbal and Alternative Medicine

Balch, James F. and Phyllis A. Balch. *Prescription for Nutritional Healing: A Practical A-to-Z Reference to Drug-Free Remedies Using Vitamins, Minerals, Herbs and Food Supplements*. Wayne, NJ: Avery Publishing Group, 2000.

Blumenthal, Mark, ed. *The Complete German Commission E Monographs: Therapeutic Guide to Herbal Medicines*. Newton, MA: Integrative Medicine Communications, 1998.

Buhner, Stephen Harrod. *Herbs for Hepatitis C and the Liver*. Pownal, VT: Storey Books, 2000.

Griffith, H. Winter, M.D. *Vitamins, Herbs, Minerals & Supplements: The Complete Guide*. New York: MJF Books, 1999.

Hobbs, Christopher. *Milk Thistle: The Liver Herb*. Santa Cruz, CA: Botanica Press, 1984.

Hobbs, Christopher. *Foundations of Health: Healing with Herbs and Other Foods*. Capitola, CA: Botanica Press, 1992.

Nutrition

Attwood, Charles R., M.D. *Dr. Attwood's Low-Fat Prescription for Kids: A Pediatrician's Program for Preventive Nutrition*. New York: Viking Press, 1995.

Baskette, Michael and Eleaneor Mainella. *The Art of Nutritional Cooking*. Upper Saddle River, NJ: Prentice Hall PR, 1998.

Margen, Sheldon. *The Wellness Encyclopedia of Food and Nutrition: How to Buy, Store and Prepare Every Fresh Food*. New York: Rebus, 1992.

The Moosewood Collective. *Moosewood Restaurant Low-Fat Favorites: Flavorful Recipes for Healthful Meals*. New York: Clarkson Potter, 1996.

Soltanoff, Jack. *Natural Healing: The Total Health and Nutritional Program*. New York: Warner Books, Incorporated, 1989.

Weil, Andrew, M.D. *Eating Well for Optimum Health, The Essential Guide to Food, Diet and Nutrition*. New York: Alfred A. Knopf, 2000.

Wood, Rebecca, et al. *The New Whole Foods Encyclopedia: A Comprehensive Resource for Healthy Living*. New York: Penguin USA, 1999.

Wellness (Emotional, Physical and Spiritual) Guides

Austin, Miriam, and Barry Kaplan (photographer). *Yoga for Wimps: Poses for the Flexibly Impaired*. New York: Sterling Publishing Company, Incorporated, 2000.

Dossey, Larry, M.D. *Reinventing Medicine, Beyond Mind-Body to a New Era of Healing*. New York: HarperCollins, 1999.

Register, Cheri. *The Chronic Illness Experience*. Center City, MN: Hazelden 1987.

Remen, Rachel Naomi, M.D. *Kitchen Table Wisdom, Stories That Heal*. New York: Riverhead Books, 1997.

Schaeffer, Rachel, Adam Mastoon (photographer), and David S. Waitz (photographer). *Yoga for Spiritual Muscles: A Complete Yoga Program to Strengthen Body and Spirit*. Wheaton, IL: Theosophical Publishing House, 1998.

Weil, Andrew, M.D. *Spontaneous Healing: How to Discover and Embrace Your Body's Natural Ability to Maintain and Heal Itself*. Ivy Books, 2000.

Other Diseases

Becker, Gretchen. *The First Year™—Type 2 Diabetes: An Essential Guide for the Newly Diagnosed*. New York: Marlowe & Company, 2001.

Bruce, Cara and Lisa Montanerelli, Ph.D. *The First Year™—Hepatitis C: An Essential Guide for the Newly Diagnosed*. New York: Marlowe & Company, 2001.

Everson, Gregory T. and Hedy Weinberg. *Hepatitis C, A Survivor's Guide*. New York: Hatherleigh Press, 1999.

Van Vorous, Heather. *The First Year™—IBS (Irritable Bowel Syndrome): An Essential Guide for the Newly Diagnosed*. New York: Marlowe & Company, 2001.

Acknowledgments

IT WAS a great pleasure to collaborate with the medical professionals who helped provide the backbone for this book. Dr. Hari Conjeevaram, an internationally renowned hepatologist and researcher, is an assistant professor at the University of Michigan in Ann Arbor. He's actively involved with the Hepatitis B Foundation, Hepatitis B International, Parents of Kids with Infectious Diseases (PKIDs) and the American Liver Foundation. Dr. Conjeevaram provided insightful counsel and wrote the foreword.

I am indebted to Dr. Sharat Misra for providing expert medical guidance and camaraderie in the challenging final months of writing this book. Dr. Misra practices gastroenterology and hepatology in New Delhi, India. He previously worked at the All India Institute of Medical Sciences in New Delhi. He is also a Fellow of the American College of Gastroenterology, and has the special talent of being able to explain complex HBV issues with simple metaphors. His insight was critical for the success of this book. I have also been able to rely on the friendship and expertise of Dr. Timothy Block, President and Chief Scientist of the Hepatitis B Foundation and Joan Block, R.N., BSN, who directs the Foundation's activities.

Thanks go to all those who gave a helping hand to this project, both directly and indirectly. Every one of the thousands of e-mails and letters of personal testimony I received over the past year has contributed in some way to the heart and soul of this book. I was privileged to receive spontaneous and generous offers of research assistance from Danielle Robinson, Maribel Quezada, Ed Mahoney, Maureen Kamischke, and Kory D'Angelo. My first-rate lineup of readers—Joel Bleifuss, Joan Block R.N., BSN, Patty Cronin, Maureen Kamischke, Pam Ladds, Tim Schellhardt, and Danielle Robinson—provided last-minute guidance, support, expertise, and wisdom.

Graham Carpio, Brent Holden, and Mary Beth Sammons provided excellent professional counsel, while Patrice Al-Saden, a nurse and liver research coordinator on the front line, was of great help at this book's naissance. Her excitement about HBV and this project was—pardon the pun—infectious. In addition, I want to acknowledge everyone involved in the design and production of this book: David Molinaro for the charts and graphs, Howard Grossman for his cover design, Pauline Neuwirth for the elegant interior pages, and Sue McCloskey at Marlowe for her attentive support.

Special thanks to my intuitive and adroit editor Matthew Lore, who wholeheartedly agreed that a medical guide could be a good read and, that with 400 million chronic cases in the world, HBV finally deserved a book of its own. Thanks to the fairy godmothers taped to my monitor: Mom, Djuna, Virginia, and Bill.

Last but not least I thank my liver for understanding that this interlude of sleep deprivation and slog was only temporary.

Index